You Are What You Wear

You Are What You Wear

WHAT YOUR CLOTHES REVEAL ABOUT YOU

JENNIFER J. BAUMGARTNER, PSYD

Da Capo
LIFE
LONG

A Member of the Perseus Books Group

Design and production by Trish Wilkinson
Set in 11 point FairfieldLTStd Light

Cataloging-in-Publication data for this book is available from the Library of Congress.

First Da Capo Press edition 2012
ISBN 978-0-7382-1520-4 (paperback)
ISBN 978-0-7382-1533-4 (e-book)

Published by Da Capo Press
A Member of the Perseus Books Group
www.dacapopress.com

Note: This book is intended only as an informative guide for those wishing to know more about health issues. In no way is this book intended to replace, countermand, or conflict with the advice given to you by your own physician. The ultimate decision concerning care should be made between you and your doctor. We strongly recommend you follow his or her advice. Information in this book is general and is offered with no guarantees on the part of the authors or Da Capo Press. The authors and publisher disclaim all liability in connection with the use of this book.

Da Capo Press books are available at special discounts for bulk purchases in the United States by corporations, institutions, and other organizations. For more information, please contact the Special Markets Department at the Perseus Books Group, 2300 Chestnut Street, Suite 200, Philadelphia, PA 19103, or call (800) 810-4145, ext. 5000, or e-mail special .markets@perseusbooks.com.

10 9 8 7 6 5 4 3 2 1

Contents

Acknowledgments

This book is dedicated to those who have the courage to make their lives better one piece at a time.

Unending appreciation and thanks to my parents for providing an example of constant service to those in need and giving me everything and anything at the sacrifice of their own needs. I love you both more than you will ever know. To my sister for selflessly helping me turn thought into word. To my brother who, by example, gave me the courage to follow my bliss. To my Grammy for her effortless style and for saying what everyone else is too afraid to say. To my love, Johnny— how lucky are we to watch each other follow our dreams—and to the Royse family for supporting us through this exciting process.

To my friends Lynn, Jennifer, Sally, Mike, and Dunbar for providing constant support, inspiration, and hours of therapy. To Rachel Simmons, Cindy Loose, and Heather Jones, whose decision to make the world a better place through their writing and willingness to help has brought me to the completion of this book. To Matt Hudson and all of those at *Psychology Today* who have given me a platform, *The Psychology of Dress,* for my dream. To the staff at Fletcher and Company, particularly Rebecca Gradinger, for their believing. To my agent,

Lucinda Blumenfeld, for her tireless work to help me stretch, realize my goals, and accomplish them. Thank you for fueling the fire! To Katie McHugh and all those at Perseus Books who have taken a chance and given me my voice.

To God for always illuminating the path for me to follow.

Introduction

⌒

The InsideOut Connection: Discovering the Psychology of Dress

Have you ever asked yourself, *What was she thinking?* after witnessing a fashion flub? Why, after losing so much weight, does a girl continue to wear her oversized sweat suit? Why does a fifty-year-old mom seem to have raided her teen daughter's closet for leggings and a mini? If you think these are merely examples of fashion ignorance or style apathy, you are underestimating the real meaning behind your clothing choices. Our clothing is a reflection of what we are thinking and what we are feeling. Often, wardrobe mishaps are simply our inner conflicts bubbling to the surface.

Clothing is an extension of who we are. Much like a turtle with its shell, we tell the world the who, the what, the where, and the when of our lives by what we wear on our backs. When we shop for and wear clothing that reflects our best self, we must consider, consciously or unconsciously, our age, size, culture, and lifestyle. We either work with these aspects of ourselves or fight against them.

For example, continuing to buy the same size clothing when you have lost or gained significant weight works against the reality of your size. Shopping at the teen clothing store when you have turned forty or buying a floor-length frock at Chico's when you are sixteen works against the reality of your age. Wearing hoodies to the office or buying embellished clothing for your job at a manufacturing plant works against the reality of your lifestyle. Your shopping may support defense mechanisms that have been reinforced over time, and you may have stopped actively noticing whether or not your clothing choices make sense for you.

Your clothes reveal more about your internal life than you may realize. Think of your closet as symptomatic. Every item in your wardrobe is the consequence of a deeper, unconscious choice. A closet full of baggy, shapeless clothes might belong to a woman who, underneath it all, is embarrassed about carrying extra weight. Perhaps she wears oversized clothes to cover the body she hates, to hide the shame she experiences, and to thwart criticism from others. Or maybe she chose these clothes because she doesn't want to lose weight, doesn't want to work out, and doesn't want to stop eating junk food, but is afraid to admit it. Maybe the closet belongs to a mom who doesn't wear nice clothes because she's pressed for time, but who might have to take notice of her failing marriage if she were less busy.

Maybe the overly youthful clothing in a closet indicates a fifty-something who finds the experience of seeing wrinkles and a couple of gray hairs just too painful to bear. Or maybe she's holding on to her past because she hasn't accomplished her goals in the present.

And some of our issues go far deeper than in these examples. We're clothing accumulators with anxiety, compulsive shoppers struggling with addiction, or frumpy dressers who suffer from depression. Our closets are windows into our internal selves. Every one of us attempts to say or hide something in the way we wear our clothes. But few of us can articulate what we're trying to express or locate the root of the pattern, the pathos.

There are all kinds of stylists who can offer your image a surface fix: a little makeup here, a pencil skirt there. That is not what I do. I am a psychologist who analyzes closets. Together, you and I will look at the patterns of your wardrobe in a way that may spark a change in how you perceive your past clothing choices and how you perceive yourself in the future, mirror optional. I "shrink" your closet down to the core of who you are. Imagine if someone could walk into your closet, look at your clothes, and diagnose an internal problem you might be having ("I can hide the body I hate in these baggy clothes"). Imagine that this person then worked with you to remove the symptoms (burn the oversized MC Hammer pants) and identify the root of the issue ("I was traumatized by bullying about my weight as a teen"), before offering a treatment ("I can learn to love my body in these trouser jeans"). As in clinical therapy, I am the objective eye that you eventually internalize. Because you are what you wear, not only can learning to identify the internal reasons for your clothing choices help you improve your wardrobe—it can change your life.

The Beginning

The day I discovered the "InsideOut" connection with clothing was the day I discovered my grandmother's closet. Looking through all of my grandmother's clothes, shoes, jewelry, and purses seemed no different than reading her journal or leafing through her photo albums. Buried in her closet were answers to the questions of who she was, where she was, who she was with, and when. Spending a day among the layers of her wardrobe became a full excavation of my grandmother's history.

The most memorable part of visiting my grandmother's closet was examining her button collection. I was dazzled by the detail and sparkle of these small objects that led to stories of her past.

I held up an amber rhinestone button. "What's this, Grammy?" I asked. She rolled it back and forth in her palm to catch the light.

"My mother, your great-grandmother, was a seamstress. This was a button from one of her very wealthy clients. A luxurious object like that during the Great Depression was a treasure."

"And this?" I asked, pointing to a large brown horn button. It belonged, she said, to the first suit she wore when she landed a job on the opening day of Macy's in New York City. "The line went around the corner. But with my tweed fur-trimmed suit and brown pumps, I was hired on the spot, Jennifer."

I handed her a large, black, onyx-faceted button. "I wore this to a sweet sixteen party when I met your grandfather. As soon as I saw him, I told my best friend I was going to marry that man."

The pile of metal and glass pieces that soon collected on my grandmother's bed became seeds out of which her story grew. I was enthralled. Whenever I visited my Grammy, I headed immediately to her closet to look for more of her.

From that day on, looking at people's wardrobes became the critical way in which I conceptualized them. And I don't mean that I made snap judgments or easy categorizations: I was looking for clues—what people wore, how they wore it, what they didn't wear, patterns of dress, what they bought, and how they organized their wardrobes—so that I could understand the whole person. My fascination with the link between external and internal human mechanisms led me to simultaneously pursue a doctoral degree in clinical psychology and to take a job as a sales associate at Ralph Lauren to pay the bills.

I'll never forget one busy holiday weekend when an attractive forty-something woman came into Ralph Lauren looking for an outfit to wear to a Christmas party. She must have tried on every item in the store before coming to the conclusion that "nothing worked" for her. Considering that everything in the store actually did work for her quite well, I knew that this general dissatisfaction had nothing to do with the clothing. After some questioning, I discovered that my customer was completely confused about her identity. Doubt and frustration poured out with her tears as she attempted to find answers. She did not know if she was old or young, mother or wife, modern or outdated, attractive or past her prime, and therefore she did not know what clothes worked for her. Although she eventually bought an outfit that day, she promptly returned it.

Psychology Meets the Closet

Even the best salesperson couldn't convince a customer like this one to make a purchase. How we dress conveys our self-concept, and this woman had deep, underlying identity confusion. I couldn't help her then, but as I began to pay more attention to the patterns of dress in the world around me, I realized that I could provide something more than a traditional wardrobe makeover. I decided to concentrate my findings into a new kind of practice. I developed what I call the "psychology of dress"—a new way of looking at dress through a psychological lens. From fellow clinicians to stay-at-home-moms, from teenage students to seventy-five-year-old grandmothers, everyone seemed to have some degree of wardrobe curiosity or confusion: What did their clothes say about them? How could they create an outfit to flatter their body? How could they curb their clothing expenses? Was there a good way to dress after times of transition? How could they identify the internal issues affecting their clothing choices?

After receiving countless requests for this psychologically informed closet makeover, I began moonlighting as a wardrobe consultant. Initially, the calls I received were from friends and family members just wanting to look better. I created and conducted my first complete InsideOut makeover on my sister, Gina, whose unchanging clothing selection echoed the stagnancy in her career and relationship pursuits. Her wardrobe hadn't been updated since middle school, and the new clothes she did own were either my castaways or clothes with tags still attached. "Gina, for God's sake, your wardrobe is in limbo. What are you waiting for?" I asked.

My sister was bored with her job and the "wimpy guys" in the dating scene. She was waiting for something bigger, and until her life magically changed, her wardrobe stayed the same.

"This isn't freakin' therapy, Jennifer," I remember her saying. "Just clean out my closet."

But I couldn't clean out her closet until I knew what, and who, Gina was dressing for in the past, present, and future. It wasn't just about the clothes: I needed to find out the type of life she had lived and was living in order to help her create the life change she desired—with a wardrobe to match. Once we had analyzed her clothes and identified her vocational, educational, and relationship goals, I could create a wardrobe that pushed her forward toward change. In this process, I realized that an inner makeover is the most essential component to an outside makeover. Without both, the change is incomplete.

The "Out" part of an InsideOut makeover, or the external, looks at the color, form, fit, and function of my clients' clothing, as well as their dressing patterns and pathology. I examine how successfully my clients shop, spend, wear, or store pieces, coordinate items, and fit their clothing to their body, how appropriately they dress for various situations, and how well their clothes are matched to their lifestyle. The "Inside" part of the makeover, or the internal, includes identifying current distress, past trauma, internal need for growth, and future goals.

My client base was soon growing as I met more and more women who could experience this connection and who invited me into their homes and closets.

When people contact me hoping to reinvent their "look," they are of-ten not prepared for the breakthrough they will actually experience. When we dig through the layers of their closet, we are really identifying and finding closure for layers of painful emotions. Talking through the stress of sorting and shopping and mirror gazing alongside someone other than yourself is therapeutic. *Acting* on these experiences through psychological techniques such as cognitive behavioral "acting as if" exer-cises, assertiveness training, and exposure activities is therapy. As a psy-chologist, I move beyond the standard closet makeover and superficial discussion of clients' self-esteem to go much deeper. They just don't real-ize it at first because they are in the safety of their closet. With all of my clients we are soon able to crack through the external shell to get to the internal "good stuff." And that's something you can't get from a stylist.

I created this book by compiling women's stories I have encountered in my life and practice; many of the women I have worked with experi-enced at least four or five of the nine most common systematic wardrobe problems detailed here. Maybe you are like Ricki, who mistakenly thinks she is a "big, ugly whale of a woman," or perhaps you have more in com-mon with Megan, who can't disentangle her work from her real life. These are the stories of women who have stripped their closets, strug-gled to answer uncomfortable questions, and worked to find answers.

At the end of each of these stories, I'll bring the analysis back to you and your closet by providing quick and easy takeaways for improving your look and your life. *You Are What You Wear* also includes a five-step wardrobe analysis—your personal tool kit for creating a healthy, balanced closet.

Our clothing is the physical representation of our perceptions, our dissatisfactions, and our desires. When we look beyond the physical to our internal workings, we can create a change at the core. Unlike change that occurs in therapy, these difficult internal examinations are softened by the lightness of the wardrobe makeover. Through this process I have witnessed people who had struggled with certain issues for years finally confront and find closure with them.

Taking care of yourself begins with self-discovery. The clothing you put on your back is an incredibly accurate indicator of what you think of yourself and your life. Cracking open the closet doors can lead to great insight. When you strive toward self-discovery, improvement often follows.

Wearing clothing that makes you feel comfortable, happy, and good about yourself really does make life better. The slightest change in your wardrobe can lead to a domino effect of adventure, discovery, and great memories. That is why I do what I do! It is so wonderful to see something that seems as insignificant as a closet makeover alter self-perception, increase self-awareness, raise self-esteem, create life goals, and encourage the pursuit of a full and well-lived life.

Swing open your closet door to discover who you are. Get rid of the clothes that don't speak to the person you have become, put on your best outfit, and walk out the door!

What's in Your Closet?
Take the Challenge

You chose to read this book for a reason. Maybe you have nothing to wear and are looking for answers. Are you experiencing wardrobe malaise? Feeling stuck when you think about making a change? These common experiences are often the result of one or more of the nine wardrobe maladies. Before any "diagnosis" can be made or a "treatment" devised, you must collect your "data," analyze that data, and then summarize your "findings."

The analysis starts with the following questions, which are designed to make you think more deeply about the patterns surrounding the way you dress. There is no one right way to approach these questions; you can answer them now or wait until after a period of observation. For now, just stick to analysis—there's no need to make any changes yet.

Past

1. Who dressed you when you were younger?
2. How did he or she dress?
3. What were you taught about getting dressed?

4. Was learning to dress a necessity, a creative process, or both?
5. When did you begin dressing yourself?
6. Did you find the process exciting?
7. Did you find the process frustrating?
8. Were you indifferent?
9. Have you suffered a wardrobe trauma, such as your dress evoking peer bullying or parent criticism?
10. How has your style changed throughout your life? For example, have you gone from punk to minimalist, tight to loose, neutrals to color?
11. What prompted these changes?
12. What has remained the same?
13. Who were your style inspirations when you were younger?
14. Have you held on to your clothes from the past?
15. What are your favorite outfits from your past and why?

Present

1. How would you describe your style now?
2. How do you feel when you get dressed?
3. Why?
4. How do you feel when you shop for clothes?
5. Why?
6. How often do you shop?
7. Why?
8. Who is your style inspiration?
9. Do you find getting dressed difficult?
10. If so, when did the difficulty start?
11. What is the most difficult part of getting dressed?
12. Do you find that you have nothing to wear?
13. Do you wear the same thing all of the time?
14. Do you wear a new outfit every day?

15. Do you dislike most of the clothes in your wardrobe?
16. Do you have a specific style that is "so you"?
17. Do you have pictures for style inspiration?
18. Do you wish you could improve the way you dress?
19. What is your favorite color?
20. Do you have that color in your wardrobe?
21. Is your style classic or trendy?
22. Traditional or modern?
23. Clean or adorned?
24. Fitted or loose?
25. Short or long?
26. Do you wear what other women in your cohort wear?
27. Have you ever tried to get help in crafting a wardrobe?
28. Is your closet full of old or new items?
29. Is your closet neatly organized or messy?
30. Is your closet empty or crammed?
31. Do you wear your clothes?
32. Do many of your clothes still have tags?
33. Do you feel that your clothes represent who you are?
34. Do you feel that your clothes flatter your body?
35. Do you feel that your clothes enhance your age?
36. Do your clothes function well with your current lifestyle?
37. What is the most common fashion mistake you make?
38. Have you tried to change this?
39. Has your style changed with a time of major transition?
40. Are you happy with this change?
41. Are you content with your current wardrobe? If so, why?

Future

1. For every decade of your life, how would you like to dress?
2. Do you have a style icon for each stage of your life?

3. What major transitions will you make in the future?
4. Do you have a wardrobe to match these changes?
5. What would your ideal wardrobe look like?
6. What changes would you like to make to your wardrobe in the future?
7. When would you like to complete the change?
8. What is keeping you from having the perfect wardrobe?
9. What goals would you like to complete in the future?
10. Have you broken these goals down into specific steps?
11. When would you like to accomplish these goals?
12. Would you like your wardrobe to facilitate this process?

The next step after this detailed analysis is summarizing your wardrobe behaviors. Identify your strengths and weaknesses. Decide what needs to change and what should stay the same.

Your diagnosis and treatment are likely to fall into one of the chapters of this book:

Chapter 1: Shop 'Til You Drop: When You Buy More Than You Need
Chapter 2: Letting Go: When Your Closet Is Overflowing
Chapter 3: Somnambulist: When You Are Bored with Your Look
Chapter 4: Body of Work: When You Avoid Mirrors
Chapter 5: Your Cover's Blown: When You Bare Too Much
Chapter 6: Adventures in Time Travel: When You Are Not Dressing for Your Age
Chapter 7: Working for It: When You Find Yourself Forever in Work Clothes
Chapter 8: It's All in the Details: When You Are Covered in Labels
Chapter 9: Getting Back to You: When You Live in Mom Jeans

Exploration is the final step of the InsideOut makeover. Choose the chapter or chapters that identify your wardrobe issues. In each chapter, you will find a detailed checklist, a case study, a psychological explanation—and solutions for your wardrobe problems that will change more than just the way you dress.

CHAPTER ONE

Shop 'Til You Drop

When You Buy More Than You Need

When Tessa called me, she had reached her limit. She briefly described her "little shopping problem" that had gotten her into a "tiny bit of trouble." As a result, she said, her closet was a mess. She needed my help to organize her many clothing purchases. I was more than happy to work with her.

I pulled up to Tessa's driveway, parked next to her shiny luxury car, and faced her sprawling colonial. Like the rest of her home, Tessa's walk-in closet was brimming with new, expensive, and designer pieces. After taking in all of this abundance, I asked Tessa what she felt the problem was.

"Well," she said, "as you can see, I have many wonderful pieces, but I am having trouble organizing them in the space and, I guess, using each piece together in order to make an outfit. I'm also wondering which of these pieces I should sell."

I nodded. "Well, we can start looking through everything to determine what stays and what goes. Selling is a great way to make the usable clothes more visible and provide room for future pieces." I was ready to begin emptying the space.

"Actually, Dr. B," Tessa said hesitantly, "I need to sell this stuff to pay off some debts. I've got plenty of room in the other closets."

And now I knew why I was really there. Like many people living above their means, Tessa had created the appearance of a lifestyle that she hadn't earned. Now she was left selling the very things that had helped her keep up appearances as she scrambled to make ends meet.

Soon the full story came tumbling out. Tessa explained that every credit card she had was now denied, her checking account was accruing overdraft fees, and the "bastard" creditors had started calling. She was upset, and her inability to organize appeared to be the superficial symptom of a much deeper issue.

Even though she had created the problem herself, Tessa's anger was misdirected at those to whom she owed money. Not only was she failing to take ownership of her inappropriate spending behaviors, but she seemed unwilling to stop. When I suggested eliminating premium cable, cutting back on the manis and pedis, and skipping the $7 coffees, Tessa looked at me as though I was asking her to give up electricity and running water.

Tessa's problem wasn't in her fashion choices, which were flawless. Her problem was that she couldn't resist the urge to shop despite being unable to afford her clothes. A habit becomes a problem when it begins to impact daily functioning, and spending her paycheck on a Burberry trench instead of her heating bill constituted a major one for Tessa.

If you are like Tessa and find that you shop when you have enough, spend money you don't have, or need to sell unworn items just to pay the bills, this chapter will show you the motivations for your behaviors and teach you the techniques to curb them. If this chapter is the one that best describes your wardrobe problem, then it's time to remove the guilt from the Gilt Groupe sales and leave the Friday nights at the mall to the teenyboppers.

Why We Buy

The predator stalks her prey for hours, anticipating just the right moment to pounce. She is hungry and ready to bring down the beast. She circles the area, assessing the landscape, seeking the perfect target. Spotting it, she locks in on it with singular focus: the clean lines, the healthy exterior, the shiny, supple skin. Who can resist the taste of victory? Ah, the hunt for handbags can be sweet.

Who hasn't had a thrilling shopping experience? Running from store to store looking for the perfect dress, shoe, or pair of jeans can be exciting. I remember a visit to Benetton years ago when I found the perfect sheath dress. It fit so well in so many places that "ah ha" moments were happening in the mirror.

That perfect shopping experience did not end in the store. I couldn't simply buy that spectacular dress in one color, not when it came in three. Sadly, my perfect sheath was not available in my size at the local store, so having convinced myself that I needed more than one of it, I continued the hunting process at home. I called another Benetton store, and then another—sold out. Finally, after scouring nearly every store in small towns all across this great country, I found my dresses. Four hours of calling was well worth the outcome.

I know well that wonderful feeling of finding something and possessing it with the swipe of a card. The urge to buy is a normal one. But the feeling of anticipation and relief associated with buying can become self-reinforcing and repetitive.

There are many psychological reasons why we are prompted to buy: we may feel anxious about other aspects of our lives, depressed

about our financial situation, or inadequate when we compare ourselves to others. Or we may just be plain bored. Whatever the reason,
buying something triggers and reinforces the brain's reward center, or
the mesolimbic system. Each time we anticipate a purchase and then
make it, we release the "feel good" chemical, dopamine, which keeps
us coming back for more. Whatever our initial psychological reasons
for going shopping, we come to know that our agitation will be immediately relieved with the dopamine-releasing purchase.

A fascinating study conducted by researchers in 2010 demon-
strated a clear connection between dopamine and compulsive shopping, also known as oniomania.* The presence of impulse control
disorders, including compulsive shopping, increased among patients
who were receiving dopamine to treat restless leg syndrome. When the
dopamine treatment was removed, the impulse disorders disappeared.

From houses to cars, knickknacks to Tupperware, clothing to jewelry, we love to buy stuff even when we don't have enough money to
pay for it! So why do we overbuy? We buy because we think we need,
we buy because we want, and we buy because we are missing something else.

Trend Chasing

We are lucky to have access to what we want whenever we want it.
We live in a time of instant gratification. With a 24/7 feed of information, we are relentlessly bombarded with ever-changing updates
about the next best thing. In response, our technological advance-
ments relieve our desires with a click of a mouse or input of a phone

---

*J. R. Cornelius, M. Tippmann-Peikert, N. L. Slocumb, C. F. Frerichs, and M.
H. Silber, "Impulse Control Disorders with the Use of Dopaminergic Agents in
Restless Legs Syndrome: A Case-Control Study," *Sleep* 33(1, 2010): 81–87.

code. The ability to quickly order from websites and shopping channels can make for mindless purchases.

How many times have we convinced ourselves that we "need" that suede ankle boot covered with zippers? Overshopping can also seem like a "necessity" if we are trying to keep up with the trends. The runways are active year-round—spring, summer, fall, winter, resort, pre-spring, pre-fall, and so on and so forth. The only way to keep up with all of the must-haves is to live, breathe, and eat shopping. One year it's the ankle boot, another year it's the above-the-knee boot. Last year it was the '80s neon punk prints and ruffles, this year it's the sculptural silhouette in patternless neutrals. Staying trendy is a full-time job.

Digging a little deeper into the standard response—that being on the cusp of fashion is exciting and fun—reveals that we follow trends to feel that we are hip and current. If everything else in our lives has fallen behind, at least we can look like we know "what's up." Being a slave to trends can hide deep insecurities, such as fear of not fitting in, fear of aging, fear of losing excitement about life, and so forth.

To avoid buying out of a perceived need that doesn't really exist, ask yourself two questions: What will be the consequences of not buying the item? And what other item do you already own that could serve as a substitute? From my experience, answers to these questions transform most potential purchases from needs into wants.

Stress Relief

Buying clothing is a true form of self-pampering. Much like a spa treatment or manicure, improving ourselves can feel like a panacea to our woes. If shopping is your form of self-soothing, your association between purchasing things and gaining stress relief will strengthen over time. According to a learning theory developed by behaviorist

B. F. Skinner, known as *operant conditioning,* if your first experience with shopping is positive, then you go online or to the mall when you need destressing in the future. Each time your stress is relieved you are positively reinforced—in other words, you will repeat this behavior. Like the hungry pigeon, anxiously increasing his pecking at the food lever in a Skinner box, the more woes you have, the more you are likely to shop. The relief you experience from clothes shopping can become an addictive remedy that leads to overspending and closet clutter.

Some people like candy, some people like trips, and some people like massages. Nothing makes me feel better than buying a piece of clothing. When I feel down, I want an outfit that will make me feel taken care of. If I have put in a hard day of work, going to the store to buy something nice with my salary feels like a well-earned reward. I receive immediate relief from my stressors. If I can't shop, my original stress is compounded by the stress I experience of not being able to shop. When I can finally get to the stores, both the stress about the situation and the agitation of delaying my shopping gratification are relieved. The negative part of my day is temporarily soothed by my shopping spree, and the shopping anticipation turns to reward.

Fitting In

We buy things to keep up, but our economy is in a shambles because people have borrowed money to pay for things they cannot afford, living well above their means. In a recent Creditcardhub.com study, data from the site's own research was combined with Federal Reserve data to examine the spending trends of the American consumer for the second quarter of the 2011 fiscal year.* This analysis

---

* CreditCardHub, "Q2 2011 Credit Card Debt Study," http://www.cardhub .com/edu/q2–2011-credit-card-debt-study (accessed November 21, 2011).

showed that consumers now carry $771.7 billion in credit card debt. Since 2009, consumers have paid their debts during the first quarter only to increase their debt during the second; in 2011 that debt increased 66 percent compared to 2010, and 368 percent compared to 2009. Even those who seemingly have enough to live comfortably spend to the point of eviction, foreclosure, and bankruptcy. If our neighbor has a one-carat ring, we want the ring with two carats. If our best friend has one Calypso caftan, then buying three caftans is even better. This cycle only ends in disappointment because someone else will always have more than we do.

When assessing your shopping wants, consider the source. Have you been watching the popular reality shows that give us a glimpse into the lives of the glitterati? Is the want really yours, or is it that of a friend, a relative, or society? Many times we shop because we have internalized "other-wants" rather than truly identified our own wants. When we are constantly told what we should have and bombarded with images of the latest and greatest products, we begin to believe that these are the things we want.

Shopping Therapy

Finally, we shop to fill a deeper hole than whatever gaps there may be in our wardrobes. We may want companionship, security, happiness, fulfillment, distractions, and diversions from ennui. Shopping can help keep us company in our isolated world, soothe painful emotions, and turn us away from what we do not want to face. Our buys offer temporary relief from something that simply won't go away.

If you are alone on a hot Saturday night, you don't feel as lonely if you are one of 751 people buying a birthstone jewelry set. Eventually, after listening to your favorite shopping network host day in and day out, you feel like you have become friends. In fact, you have become part of the shopping network family. They send you schedules, flyers, and even birthday cards! You now belong to a friendly club that never judges or requires anything of you, but you somehow always feel obligated to give back and buy. How can I resist making a purchase when David Venable is hosting? Impossible!

Overbuying clothing and accessories can often indicate a dissatisfaction we have about ourselves but are unable to resolve internally. When we buy at the mall, we hope these external trappings will fix our dissatisfaction. Although our new wardrobe pieces may temporarily fix our perceived deficit, this effect is short-lived, and we must soon head to the store for another attempt.

If you feel that you are not smart enough, pretty enough, successful enough, or just enough in general, buying stuff can help disguise those flaws. Who will notice that you aren't all that if you are wearing a fabulous outfit? Who will notice that you have a crappy job when you are wearing the latest trend? Who will notice your aging face when you are bedecked with your newest rhinestone necklace?

When we are unhappy with the life we *have,* we often create the life we *want* through our trappings. With all of our new stuff, we can set the scene for our ideal life even if it is not really there. Our fancy cars, big homes, plush furniture, and designer shoes are merely optical illusions that hide the financial strain, the family conflict, and the general emptiness.

Wanting to buy something becomes problematic when we don't have the resources to buy it, we don't have the room to store it, and we never have the occasion to use it. To experience a state of want is in actuality to experience a state of anxiety. To resolve this anxiety, we can either allow ourselves to experience the discomfort without acting on it or release the anxiety through buying things. The shopping difficulties begin when we continue to buy to calm ourselves without ever experiencing and working through our anxiety.

The drive to possess, consume, and outdo is reminiscent of the donkey chasing the dangling carrot. No matter how hard he tries, he will never get the carrot dangling just out of reach. When we overspend and overbuy, we are often trying to find fulfillment that cannot be achieved through material acquisitions.

Are You OverBuying? A Checklist

- ❏ Do you think about buying things most or all days?
- ❏ Do you shop to celebrate or as a reward?
- ❏ Do you shop to cope with a problem or because you are bored?
- ❏ Do you find that you experience anxiety before you shop, followed by relief after you shop?
- ❏ After you buy an item, does the excitement quickly wear off?
- ❏ Do you feel guilty about your purchases or hide them from others?
- ❏ Have you ever told yourself that you will never buy again?
- ❏ Do you wish that you had the items that your friends and family have?
- ❏ Do you feel inadequate when someone has something and you don't?
- ❏ Is your shopping causing short-term relief and long-term problems?
- ❏ Did you read this chapter because it described you?
- ❏ Do you find yourself putting aside sleep, friends, work, or other activities to shop in stores or online?
- ❏ When you shop, do you often find that you spend more or buy more items than you had intended?
- ❏ Do you buy things you normally would not because they are on sale?
- ❏ Even after you try to stop, do you still buy?
- ❏ Do sales associates know you on a first-name basis?

❏ Are you receiving regular email alerts for sales, promotions, and in-store events?

❏ Do you have saved accounts for television and online stores?

❏ Do you have a shopping wish list? Once you buy a wish list item, do you immediately focus on another?

❏ Do you have duplicate items in your closet?

❏ Are there still tags on many of your clothes and accessories?

❏ Do you find that your closet is not big enough for all your stuff?

❏ Do you feel that you should never wear the same outfit twice?

❏ Have your friends and family commented on your shopping behaviors?

❏ Do you find that you cannot afford to pay your bills?

❏ Are you anxious about consumer debt?

❏ Is the majority of your income spent on acquiring items?

❏ Do you find that you engage in avoidance behaviors surrounding debt (not paying your bills, changing your number to deter creditors, throwing away your mail, and so on)?

❏ Do you ever think, fearing that your debt may become too large for you to shop one day, that you "might as well get it now"?

❏ Do you ask others to buy for you or borrow money from them?

If you answered yes to most of these questions, your shopping habits are likely unmanageable. When behaviors cause great distress or result from unhealthy internal motivations, it is time to make a change.

Case Study: Why Tessa Worked for Clothes That Didn't Work for Her

My primary goal for Tessa was to make the connection between her stuff and her emotional motivation to buy it. I let her think that we were just looking through her clothes, making outfits, and removing items for sale, but in the process we would find the internal reasons for her out-of-control spending.

We dug into the clothes to find the triggers for Tessa's shopping behavior. The best way to deal with compulsive behaviors, even those manifested in the closet, is to use a model of treatment for serious addictive behaviors. Tessa and I would need to identify the triggers for her shopping behaviors, find replacement behaviors, remove enablers, create an emergency plan of action, eliminate the means to pay for the items, and generate a support network to help her through the first and most difficult few weeks.

So we started the cleaning process by throwing all of the clothes on the bed. I hoped that if Tessa could see all of the items she already owned laid out before her, she might have difficulty justifying future purchases. We separated her clothing into two piles: those that she could keep and those that needed to be given away or thrown away.

"Tessa, you have done a great job sorting through the good stuff and the bad stuff," I told her when we completed this step. "We have definitely identified what you can sell for extra cash, and I think you will get a nice amount for it. Let's try to make outfits from the pieces you purchased."

We separated the clothes into two primary categories, the tops and the bottoms. As Tessa separated the clothes on her bed, I noticed that most items had tags still attached. I also noticed that, although still expensive, the prices of these items had been marked down. Now I had some method to Tessa's madness.

Observation 1: Tessa did not buy pieces out of need. If she did, she would have had outfits. She bought pieces impulsively and without awareness of the bigger picture in her closet. The pieces in her closet were highly disjointed.

Observation 2: Tessa did not wear most of what she had. The pieces in her closet were being treated like museum artifacts rather than wearable clothing.

Observation 3: Finally, Tessa spent money on things that were on sale. I hypothesized that she needed the discount—and I use that term very loosely—to ease the guilt of her spending.

"It's Too Nice to Wear"

While throwing all of her items on the bed from her closet, Tessa tried her best to conceal the tags still attached to each item. The clothes she was wearing that day—ratty oversized jeans, a rumpled tank, and a lumpy bra—gave me a clue that this was what she usually wore, not her attractive clothing.

"Tessa, why haven't you worn any of this stuff?" I was expecting to hear what I usually hear: *I hate my body. I'm too fat. I'm out of shape. I don't have a reason to.* Instead, Tessa said that her well-tailored, classic clothes were "too good to wear." She was afraid that she might "ruin or waste an outfit" if she didn't stick to her scrubby everyday wear.

Why would Tessa buy clothes that she would never wear? Underneath everything, Tessa felt guilty about her choices. Not wearing the items she so desperately craved was a form of self-punishment. She had already rewarded herself with the "bad" purchase; therefore, she could not reward herself again by wearing it. Additionally, as most of us do with behaviors that are bad for us, Tessa would swear that each time would be the last time. She was saving purchases in her closet just in case that turned out to be true. If she had to eventually stop shopping, at least she still had those pristine items she could enjoy.

Before I left for the day, Tessa and I looked through the "too good to wear" pieces and began to stratify them. We separated them into four categories:

Level 4: Formal
Level 3: Night out
Level 2: Office
Level 1: Weekend casual

I asked Tessa to move any outfit she would usually consider an upper level of clothing to a lower level. For example, she would normally wear a nice pair of jeans, sandals, and a tank for a night out; now this outfit was moved down to "weekend casual." Her flirty dress that she had been saving for formal wear was demoted to "night out." This intervention prevented Tessa from underdressing and ensured that she wore her special clothing. We would later take inventory and fill the holes in Tessa's wardrobe in a way that was consistent with her lifestyle, the idea being to make sure that no clothing in her closet ever again remained unworn.

Looking for Triggers

Now Tessa needed to analyze what prompted her to shop. I asked her to *observe without making changes* for one week. She could shop, buy, and browse as much as she desired, but for that week she had to document what was happening in her life right before she felt the urge. I could then analyze the data to find Tessa's emotional triggers.

In a week's time, I returned to Tessa's house prepared to examine her observations every time she shopped. During a five-day period, Tessa had shopped three times and recorded everything that happened that day prior to shopping.

"When you left, I was feeling proud of myself for giving away so much of my stuff, and I figured I was going to make some pretty good money from it, so I decided to treat myself. I woke up early the next morning and went to Neiman's. They were having a sale on some Michael Kors stuff . . . and there you have it."

"Good, Tessa, you made some connections here. You were feeling good, and you wanted a reward. Okay, what about the second time?"

"Well, that night when I took my purchases home, I felt a bit guilty about what I had done. Oh yeah, and the rent that was due didn't help either. So, as usual, I promised myself that that shopping trip would be my last. Then I somehow convinced myself that I didn't officially make it my last, so I would need an official one. Hence the second shopping trip."

"So you are on your second trip, and? . . ."

"I went with the goal of making this my last trip for a long time, so I needed to make it a special one. I bought these designer shoes that I have had my eye on forever. Lucky for me, I had a coupon, so it could have been worse."

"I can understand wanting to mark something special, but it didn't end there, did it, Tessa?"

"Well, the last one was totally not my fault. On Thursday, my coworker wanted to celebrate her birthday, so after work she invited me to go shopping with her. She was so excited, so I really couldn't help myself. I saw these two adorable dresses from Zara that would work really well with my new shoes, but then I needed a belt to work with the dresses and the shoes, so I headed on over to Saks to find a matching belt. Instead, I decided on some really cool leather pants. Thought it was something I should have, and maybe a bit more practical than the belt."

"Tessa, what are you noticing here in your shopping journal? What are your triggers?"

She responded that she usually bought when she experienced very positive or very negative emotions, and that she felt better about buying because her items, although still expensive, were almost always on sale.

Emotional Highs and Lows

We've all heard of emotional eating. There's also such a thing as emotional shopping. In moderation, neither of these activities is harmful, but in excess both can have serious consequences. By temporarily creating positive emotions, these activities can prevent a true examination of our real feelings and negatively impact all areas of our lives. And I haven't even gotten to the aftermath of pain and guilt! The cycle is self-reinforcing. We shop to feel good, we feel good for a bit, then we feel bad, only to shop to try to feel good again.

The shared experience, the accessibility, the affordability, and the reinforcing messages make our shopping behavior all the more enticing. Who do we know who doesn't shop? Shopping is a collective experience. Sometimes we shop alone, but alongside our peers, and sometimes we shop with a partner. And when we shop with someone, we may buy more than we had intended, especially if we are men.*

In and of itself, Tessa's sale-scouring behavior was a superficial issue; the deeper reason for her spending would be far more difficult to identify and remedy. Often we feel emotional experiences as either an

---

*D. Kurt, J. J. Inman, and J. J. Argo, "How Friends Promote Consumer Spending," *Journal of Marketing Research* 38(August 2011): 741–754.

overwhelming surge or a gnawing emptiness. When I examined Tessa's shopping journal, I saw that she experienced both kinds of emotion.

"When I am excited about doing something well or about what is happening in the day, I want to feel even better, and shopping is a way to increase that high." During times of positive emotion, Tessa wanted to amplify those feelings with her favorite friend, the shopping cart.

"When I'm depressed, it is just the opposite. I get so down that I shop to feel better. I get a little lift, but it's never enough, so I have to shop again." When Tessa felt the emptiness of sadness, the clothes, shoes, and jewelry would fill her up—for a while.

Tessa also noticed that her wardrobe was not cohesive. Her clothing choices arose out of various emotional states, so many of the pieces did not fit together. During these times of highs and lows, Tessa bought pieces that she did not need and that did not match anything else in her wardrobe. When she wore these fragmented pieces, they reminded her of the difficult time when she bought them. Therefore, she had never worn most of her clothes.

Hearing her speak of her emotional highs and lows, I imagined a line graph with peaks and troughs. When Tessa was sad and her trough plummeted below baseline (aka the status quo or general functioning), her shopping pulled her up to the baseline. When she was excited, Tessa's peaks were above baseline, and shopping pulled the peaks up even more. What Tessa did not see was that these shopping highs did not last long. And after the high wore off, Tessa felt worse. Guilt from overspending never is good for the psyche.

A Great Deal

Tessa often took weekly shopping trips to scour the stores for sale items. Unfortunately, a sale price does not make an item purchase-worthy. She would bring home bags of clothing that included multiples of the same item, unneeded accessories, and clothing that didn't fit with her lifestyle or any other clothes in her wardrobe.

When I asked Tessa why she bought all of these items, she stated, "Well, I had to—they were on sale!" Tessa needed to dig a bit deeper, and after much discussion, I helped her see that the sale price tag took the edge off of the purchase. It removed some of the aftershock and guilt when she was left alone in her room to tackle her ever-mounting debt. But sales are worthwhile only if they save us money, which presumes that we are buying items we actually *need* at a reduced cost. Not so with Tessa.

Breaking this habit can be difficult because it does have immediate short-term benefits. When Tessa went out looking for a good deal, she always found one and was therefore able to justify buying unnecessary items. Unfortunately, she did not consider the long-term disadvantages. The amount spent buying unnecessary items on sale ultimately equals the price of wearable key pieces, which may not be on sale.

Breaking the Cycle

Stores make it so easy to shop these days. Gone are the three-week trips by horse and buggy to get a pound of sugar and some ribbon. We can buy at home or just around the corner. Even when we're not shopping, commercials, magazines, online ads, promotions, coupons, and so forth encourage us to be thinking about it. With all that the world of stuff has to offer, it seems like we would be crazy to pass up on the opportunity to acquire it.

"Tessa, do you realize that the temptation to shop is all around you?" I remarked. "No wonder it is so difficult to cease and desist." I explained to Tessa that if she really wanted to change, her environment would also need to be changed. We discussed the difference between changes that would be reasonable and changes that would be just setting her up for failure.

Once she made the connection between her shopping and her emotions, she was able to prepare a plan for the next crisis. This plan included finding effective replacements for shopping that would not burn a hole in her wallet and that would have long-term benefits.

Tessa started by alerting her friends and family that she was on a shopping "live-it" ("diet" is such an awful word). She would love to shop with them, she told them, but she was unable to buy until she had changed her compulsive behaviors into healthy behaviors and her budget was repaired. To do this, she agreed to leave her wallet in her car before any shopping outing.

Tessa also agreed to complete a monthly budget that allowed a small cash amount to be used specifically for shopping. I wanted to decrease her compulsive behavior, but completely forbidding her to shop would probably have caused Tessa to binge-shop.

Tessa was allowed, however, to *damage-free shop* when she found herself in a state of shopping emergency. This is a technique that takes the edge off a desire to shop by providing some relief. Tessa wrote down all of the items she wanted, including the price and the order information. A week later, she could return to her list and discover that her craving to buy these items had probably passed. Being a lover of fashion, Tessa had many fashion magazines and frequented online fashion sites. After tabbing, circling, and filing away her must-have items, she could go through the process of craving, stalking, and conquering her fashion desires in a safe way.

Finally, Tessa was placed on a "no-sale" restriction until we had fully cleaned and organized her closet. She would avoid stores having sales, and she let her friends and family know that she was not allowing herself to buy anything on sale. To help her break her bargain shopping habit, I suggested to Tessa that she calculate her monthly spending on sale clothing and the number of times she wore those items. From these figures, Tessa calculated the actual amount she spent on each article per wear. For example, if Tessa had spent $80 on a dress but had worn it only two times, the dress was actually costing her $40 per wear. If Tessa had worn the same dress twenty times, the dress would cost $4 per wear. This calculation was shocking to Tessa, who, after five years, had clothing in her closets still in bags with the tags attached.

After a month of shopping journaling, alerting her friends to the changes she was making, creating a budget, and engaging in guilt-free shopping, Tessa reported that she was able to weather the cravings to buy.

"I still have this urge to buy, but I have alternatives that feel like I am actually shopping. It's nice to actually experience my emotions rather than enhance or dull them. When I am happy, I am happy. When I am sad, I can fully feel the sadness."

There is nothing wrong with buying clothing to make yourself feel better. If anyone believes in the power of shopping and dressing well, it is me! There is something wrong, though, when an inanimate object replaces the expression of true emotion, halts the necessary process of confrontation, and blocks the path to resolution.

Thanks to the no-sale restriction, Tessa eventually had enough extra spending money at the end of each month to contribute to her savings, go out to dinner with friends, host dinner parties, and pursue her love of travel. As Tessa came to appreciate the long-term benefits of only buying items that she needed or loved, we lifted the no-sale restriction. I am happy to report that Tessa no longer frequents the early bird sales or drives to the middle of nowhere to hunt for the latest bargain at outlet stores, and she even has managed to take the sale postcards that arrive in her mailbox and drop them straight into the recycling bin.

For Tessa, finding social support was the best cure for a bad shopping habit and bad clothing choices. She did not succeed overnight in making these changes; it took much time and dedication. The result, though, was a closet filled with well coordinated pieces, which had a positive and uplifting effect on her.

At the end of the InsideOut makeover, Tessa, like Dorothy in *The Wizard of Oz,* realized that everything she needed was right under her nose. She did not need to run to the mall to find more—she already had a closet filled with beautiful items. She just needed to learn how to wear them. She also learned that the emotional experience she so desperately sought was already inside of her, free of charge.

Your Turn

Shopping without means *is* a problem. When the thought of want moves you to action, the compulsive reinforcements take hold. Each time you buy, your desire to buy again grows.

Tessa bought without wearing, bought during sales, and bought with unchecked emotion. If you are like Tessa, you are not alone. You can help yourself, but if you find that you can't do that on your own, professional help is available. Remember, even though your closet is full, you may still be empty. There is no greater investment you can make than the investment you make in yourself.

Spending Spiral

Do you also use clothing to fill an emotional void and soothe yourself? Are you plagued by shopping patterns that simply add to a wardrobe of mismatched and unloved pieces? When you wear your clothes, do they remind you of loves lost, jobs terminated, or life disappointments?

You may not be aware that you are using clothing to quiet your emotions. Compulsive shopping is like any other addiction. The urge is overwhelming, the short-term effect soothes, and the long-term effect creates guilt, anxiety, and, in this case, a useless wardrobe. Whether you have a shopping pattern that is clinically compulsive (severe enough that it warrants professional treatment) or just a mild case of "shopping away the blues," you can use an addiction treatment model to stop filling your closet with stuff!

You must first identify your shopping patterns, beginning with triggers to your behaviors. As with any addiction treatment, identifying the triggers of your compulsive behavior can eventually lead to effective treatment. Although many people shop when they are sad, it is also possible that you shop to celebrate, or maybe you shop because you simply have extra money to spend. Ask yourself why you are buying the clothes that you buy: are they necessities or mindless purchases? At this stage, it is unnecessary to change your behavior, only to make note of it.

Once you have identified your triggers, however, it's time to begin to change the behavior. One of the most helpful ways to stop a behavior is to recognize the urge to engage in it and then engage in new replacement behaviors instead, such as socializing with friends, getting some exercise, journaling, watching a movie, or taking a bubble bath. Everyone has different replacement behaviors they prefer, so take the time to find yours. When you do, your shopping will no longer be a dysfunctional treatment, but a treat!

Resist the Sale

Not only did Tessa not wear her clothes, but she never paid full price for them. I had to diagnose her with *sale insanity*. The first step in curing a sale obsession is identifying whether your dedication to getting a deal is problematic. When you are buying clothes because you love them and use them, bargain hunting is worth the time, effort, and money you expend. But if you are not using these items, or not feeling fabulous in them, then all of the resources you expended are lost without any return.

To reframe the way you think about sale shopping, look at filling your closet the same way you would a savings account. Buying something at a discounted price does not necessarily mean that you have made a good investment. To actually save money and increase the amount that you have in your account, you must wear whatever you buy, and love it too. If you don't wear it or love it, you have lost money from your account even if you got a "great deal."

Another more concrete method for changing how you think about sale shopping is to calculate your actual expense per wear of an item. As happened with Tessa, this technique helps you put your spending habits into perspective.

With the advent in this country of shopping warehouses, discounted superstores, and outlets, more and more people are exposed to more and more stuff. All of this stuff is purchased guilt-free owing to the discounted prices. Research has shown that people leave these stores having bought more items than they intended to buy because they got such a "great deal." This is similar to the findings from food consumption studies spearheaded by Dr. Brian Wansink of Cornell University. His team consistently found that, the more food participants saw, the more food they would eat; the more food there was on their plate, the more food they ate from it.* True to human nature, we always consume what's in front of us.

----

* B. Wansink, *Mindless Eating: Why We Eat More Than We Think* (New York: Bantam Dell, 2006).

Europeans do it best when it comes to bargain shopping—they don't. Instead, they buy fewer things of greater quality, style, and cost. I can clearly recall my *professeur de française* stating that she did not understand the American method for choosing *habiliments*. A French woman, she insisted, only needs a black cashmere turtleneck, dress pants, jeans, a white collared shirt, a Hermes scarf, a trench, a pair of flat shoes, and a pair of heels. Cost is immaterial because, even though French women purchase these items from the highest end, they can endure a lifetime.

Quick Tips for Stopping the Shopping Cycle

If you are trying to battle your shopping compulsions, whether they impair your functioning to a degree that requires a clinical intervention or fall within "normal" limits, putting an end to the cycle can feel impossible. The urge to shop can be overwhelming, and the relief you experience each time you buy becomes stronger than your guilt and fear of debt. The benefits from stopping compulsive shopping behaviors must be greater than the relief you gain from continuing them.

To battle shopping impulses, you must begin by reducing those impulses. When you shop compulsively, your emotions are bringing on knee-jerk reactions: *I feel nervous (upset, unfulfilled), and now I will shop away the pain.* Emotion leads to action. To slow down or halt this process, your emotion should lead to *thought,* which should then lead to action. Making room for a logical and thoughtful consideration of emotion and future action can be the critical piece in reducing your shopping sprees.

If you are among the many who shop without need, means, or a clear head, the following shopping techniques can bring relief to your mind and your wallet.

Shopping without: Who doesn't love to look at clothes, feel clothes, try on clothes, or see new clothing styles? Clothes are pieces of art on hangers. When you need to control your shopping impulses and are not allowing yourself to spend, you may still feel the urge to shop. *Shopping without* means shopping without your wallet. No credit cards, no cash, no check, no nothing! Now, to hard-core shoppers, shopping without your wallet handy may seem like a slow form of torture. It may feel somewhat painful at first, but it will stretch out the time between when you feel the need to buy and when you buy an item having put actual thought and consideration into the purchase.

After shopping without your wallet, come home with your mental list of "must have" items. Then examine your real closet needs: are these items just impulse wants, or would they be real investments in the wardrobe you already own? You may find that 10 percent of the items on your shopping-without list actually make it home.

Texas hold 'em: When you use my *Texas hold 'em* technique, go shopping, find all of the items you really must have, and then put them on hold. Keep them on hold until the shopping day is over or the close of the next day. While the items are on hold, go home and review what you have and see whether your collection already includes items that could be substituted for the hold items. Decide on your hold items only after carefully reviewing what you have and what you need.

Time limit: The *time limit* technique forces you to face your anxiety when you are not able to buy, to sit with that anxiety, and then to make a decision based on thought rather than emotion. Each time you are able to conquer your anxiety about not shopping, you learn that the feeling to shop impulsively will decrease. If you are able to wait out the need to buy for a week or a month, reassess whether you still want the item, and decide that the answer is yes, then you have permission to buy it.

Own it: I used the *own it* technique when I worked in retail. Oddly enough, when I was surrounded by clothing and could easily buy the best and newest clothing with a hefty discount, the desire to buy went down the drain. I hated the mall, despised shopping, was sick of clothing, threw away catalogs, and bought almost nothing. I always felt that the store was my closet and that I could technically have anything I wanted in that big beautiful closet. The impulsivity and the forbidden fruit quality of shopping disappeared. When I felt like I owned it, I didn't want it.

You don't have to work in retail to try this technique. If you have a picture of the item you want, post it on a mirror where you can see it every day. This kind of super-saturation with an item often leads to satiety. I have been known to visit items that I love but may not have any business buying, including Manolo Blahnik shoes, an Asscher cut engagement ring, and a diamond-encrusted Cartier Tank Americaine. The Internet is also a great way to bombard yourself with an item before you actually buy it. After many visits to your virtual shopping cart, you may find that your interest in downloading this financial death trap from the Internet disappears.

Registration frustration: The Internet makes impulsive shopping quick and easy. No driving, no parking, no trying on, no crowds, no lines, and no closing time. You can shop in the comfort of your own home at 3:00 AM with your hair full of curlers and a tub of Nutella and a spoon close by. This no-hassle shopping can be extremely dangerous for anyone with a serious shopping problem.

Giving up shopping is never easy in a time of easy access. When I foolishly gave up my out-of-control shopping behavior for Lent, I knew that I had to tackle the Internet problem. Having pre-registered accounts at Ralph Lauren, Neiman Marcus, Saks, Burberry, Banana Republic, Tory Burch, and Nordstrom was not going to make it easier to do that. So what did I do? I disabled my accounts, creating *registration frustration* for myself.

Clicking directly from "Shopping Cart" to "Place Your Order" should not be so easy. When I had to take the time to type in all of my information, I found that I was more likely to stretch out the time between emotion and action and take more time to think about the necessity of my purchase. Even after Lent was over, my shopping impulses were cured . . . temporarily.

Mindful purchasing: Impulsive behavior is often mindless behavior. Another way to change the way you shop is to take the time to actually think about it through *mindful purchasing.* You can become mindful or aware of what you are feeling before you shop; where, when, and why you shop; what you feel when you shop; what you feel after you shop; and when you are likely to shop again. Mindful purchasing is also another way to assess your actual need for a new wardrobe item, to determine what you already have in order to know what you might need now, and to differentiate between need and want.

It is not easy for me to sit still, and it is certainly not easy for me to "sit with my thoughts." Sometimes you just don't want to hear yourself. As part my training to become a psychologist, I needed to learn how to facilitate a client's ability to reach some level of mindfulness, and that required that I become mindful myself. After much resistance I finally caved in, and soon I had realized the benefits to meditation, relaxation, deep breathing, and journaling as I cultivated the here-and-now awareness that comes with mindful practices. Becoming mindful of my emotions and resultant behaviors was essential to putting a lid on my shopping insanity. Now I think through my purchases before swiping the credit card.

The Basics:
Shopping for Clothing Successfully

Sometimes overbuying results not from a love for shopping, an obsession with trends, or internal struggle. You may simply be uncertain about how to craft a wardrobe out of all the pieces you own. If your wardrobe is filled with pieces that don't easily mix and match, your only choice in a fashion emergency is to buy something new that will work in that moment.

Closets can be filled with purchases from "I've got nothing to wear" emergencies that often do not work with other items in your closet. This shopping habit has a self-reinforcing effect. The more you buy in the heat of the moment, the more you will need. According to Gestalt theory, the whole should be greater than the sum of the parts. Even if your closet includes fabulous pieces, the whole of your wardrobe will fail if the pieces are disjointed from each other. Learning to craft a cohesive wardrobe out of multifunctional pieces can cure anyone of the impulse to over-shop under pressure.

Some of the best tips for creating a wardrobe can come from home decor. The workhorses of a home—the chairs, tables, and couches—should be proportionate to the dimensions of the space, should have a simple classic form, should fit the general style of the other items, and should have a color scheme that works with the other pieces. Accessories like pillows, artwork, and rugs should make the room pop and can more easily be changed to reflect trends. The main furniture pieces should serve as the canvas, while accessories serve as the paint on that canvas.

As a general rule for your wardrobe, choose classic "workhorses" such as a black or camel suit, dark straight-leg jeans, a sheath dress, or tweed pants in a flattering cut and solid color. Steer clear of crazy patterns and embellishments of glitter, rhinestones, tassels, and so forth. Avoid the trends when buying wardrobe staples and get creative instead in buying accessories, such as shoes, belts, scarves, and jewelry. Here is where you can experiment with color, fabrics, beading, and patterns.

When you have chosen your classic wardrobe items thoughtfully, you'll see that they can easily transition between various occasions, be adjusted for the time of day and the temperature, and accommodate any level of dress. Recall that we categorized Tessa's wardrobe into four levels:

Level 4: Formal
Level 3: Night out
Level 2: Office
Level 1: Weekend casual

You may have fewer than four levels, or more, but this general wardrobe hierarchy can help you identify the pieces that easily transition throughout the levels (the classics) and those that are specific to a level (specialty items).

Start by picking one item in your closet, such as a white buttondown. Mix and match the piece with other things in your closet.

Level 4 *Formal:* wear the shirt with a tuxedo pant or long satin skirt, strappy shoes, and hair pulled back in a low chignon
Level 3 *Night-out:* wear the shirt with a fitted skirt, mini, or formal shorts, platform pumps, and hair down in waves

Level 2 *Office:* wear the shirt under a strapless scoop-neck
sheath with a blazer or cardigan, or with wide leg
trousers or a pencil skirt, kitten heels or feminine
loafers, and hair worn straight or in a low ponytail

Level 1 *Weekend casual:* wear the shirt with a faux fur vest,
skinny jeans, and riding boots, and hair held back
by a headband

From this exercise, you can easily see that the white button-down
is indeed a wardrobe workhorse, a keeper. No matter what level
you're dressing at, this item always looks appropriate and can work
with many other pieces in your wardrobe. Now, let's say you are shopping for new pieces to add to your wardrobe and can't decide between
a long strand of pearls and the thigh-high leather stiletto boots. Try re-
peating the exercise.

Level 4 *Formal:* wear with a tuxedo pant or long satin skirt,
strappy shoes, and hair pulled back in a low chignon—
you could wear the pearls as a tiered choker and fasten
a diamond brooch to the strands.

Level 3 *Night-out:* wear with a fitted skirt, mini, or formal
shorts, platform pumps, and hair down in waves—you
could tie the pearls into a knot at the bottom or wear
them against your neck and hanging down your back,
and you could wear the thigh-high boots instead of
platform pumps.

Level 2 *Office:* wear under a strapless scoop-neck sheath with a
blazer or cardigan, or with wide leg trousers or a pencil
skirt, kitten heels or feminine loafers, and hair straight
or in a low ponytail—you could wear pearls full length.

Level 1: Weekend casual: wear with a faux fur vest, skinny jeans, and riding boots, and hair held back in a headband—you could wrap the pearls into a layered bracelet.

The pearls can work at every level, but the thigh-high boots would work only at Level 3. Now the choice is obvious!

To Have and to Hold

If, like Tessa, you have beautiful clothes in your closet and are not wearing them, you're committing the most egregious fashion crime. Wear the wonderful things in your closet—the special occasion you were saving them for is now! And if you know you are not going to wear them, give the clothes to someone who will.

The meaning in life is in finding what we have to offer others. We are all put on this planet with certain resources, our gifts and talents, to make the lives of others easier. If you have something to give someone else, give it. That goes for wardrobes too! If you have wonderful clothes in your closet that you have not used, give them away.

Each time you purchase something, *always* give something else away. This accomplishes two things: (1) You increase someone else's happiness, and (2) you have an opportunity to take stock of what you already have in your closet, to remove things you do not wear, and to make space for new items. This intervention ensures that you never have more than you have space to hold. You can practice giving away not only your clothes this way, but also all the items you have.

⌐⌐

Life feels better when we eliminate the unnecessary and surround ourselves with the things that do not simply collect dust but have meaning for us.

A Note on
Compulsive Buying Disorder

Those who continue to buy regardless of the negative impact on their lives have taken shopping to a clinical level. True compulsive buying disorder (CBD) is also known as oniomania. CBD occurs in well below 10 percent of the population, primarily in females, with average onset of late teens or twenties. Although the prevalence and incidence of this disorder have increased in the last few decades, research and clinical practice to treat it have not matched the need. Unfortunately, although this chronic disorder was recognized in the early twentieth century and has been found worldwide, especially in countries with products to buy en masse, it remains unknown and undefined to this day.*

Compulsive buying disorder begins with the buildup of a feeling of tension or anxiety before making a purchase. The purchase then releases this feeling. This behavior becomes impulsive, excessive, and repetitive, and the pattern of anxiety and release through shopping leads to distress, impairment, and financial problems and interferes with familial, social, and occupational functioning. This impulse control disorder is invasive and extremely difficult to control because the release of negative emotions through shopping is initially soothing and seems to override the long-term consequences.

---

* D. W. Black, "A Review of Compulsive Buying Disorder," *World Psychiatry* 6(1, February 2007): 14–18.

CBD seems to run in families and has a neurobiological cause. It often occurs with other psychological disorders, so making a separate clinical diagnosis or sorting out symptoms of other disorders is often difficult. Mood, anxiety, substance use, eating, impulse control, obsessive-compulsive behavior, and personality disorders often occur with CBD. Many compulsive buyers are also compulsive hoarders. Treatment is difficult, but antidepressant medication and cognitive behavioral therapy groups have shown some effectiveness.*

---

* Ibid.

CHAPTER TWO

Letting Go

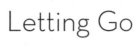

When Your Closet Is Overflowing

The magnetic closures barely hold as your closet doors are pushed to capacity. Shoes piled on the floor topple underneath all the dirty clothes that no longer fit in the hamper. The area is now brimming with bags and boxes of new items, still waiting to be worn. Above, metal racks bend under the weight of outdated blazers, mismatched suits, nubby tops, ripped jeans, holiday sweaters, Halloween costumes, and once-worn bridesmaid dresses. Like New York real estate, closet space is at a premium, but isn't that what under the bed is for?

In our country, clutter is king. We continually bring new items into our households without removing old items to accommodate them, which creates a home filled to capacity and beyond. Since 1970, home sizes in the United States have increased from 1,500 square feet to between 2,000 and 2,500 square feet.* Today many

---

* US Census Bureau, "Median and Average Square Feet of Floor Area in New Single-Family Houses Completed by Location," http://www.census .gov/const/C25Ann/sftotalmedavgsqft.pdf (accessed November 26, 2011).

homeowners have a two-car garage in which they cannot fit a vehicle because it serves as a storage area. Whatever does not fit in the home is packed away in a rental storage unit. Consider a popular weight loss theory as a parallel: if calories in exceed calories out, weight is gained; if calories in are fewer than calories out, weight is lost; and if calories in equal calories out, weight is maintained. Is this not true of our living spaces? Our bodies may stretch, but unfortunately for our homes, our closets do not!

Are you guilty of square footage theft? The two behaviors that lead to excess possessions are buying and keeping. While Chapter 1 addressed acquiring stuff, this chapter examines why we keep it. Many of us have things that we "just can't give away." This desire to keep things can reach unhealthy levels, impacting our social, occupational, and physical health.

Not everyone who collects and keeps stuff is a hoarder. Although the term *hoarder* is thrown around quite casually in the media and in our daily conversations, compulsive hoarding is actually a clinical diagnostic term, not to be confused with the common term *clutter bug*. Compulsive hoarding syndrome is a serious psychological illness that ranges in severity and affects less than 1 percent of the population.[*] It is characterized by an "excessive collection of items with the inability to discard them." This disorder is extremely difficult to treat and is often accompanied by other disorders, such as obsessive-compulsive disorder, eating disorders, and dementia.

Whether you are a true hoarder or, more likely, a person who has accumulated clutter, you are impacted by the contents of your space. The aesthetic of your space both reflects and determines your mood. When

---

[*] Mayo Clinic, "Hoarding: Definition," http://www.mayoclinic.com/health /hoarding/DS00966 (last modified May 25, 2011).

I walk into a cluttered space, I feel that I have no room to spread out, physically, emotionally, or mentally. Conversely, when I am in a space that is empty and austere, I feel exposed and vulnerable. The anchors of comfort, such as a soft blanket or a couch full of pillows, are not there; the space feels cold, clinical, and impersonal. The key to a comfortable home or a successful wardrobe is finding the balance between fullness and emptiness. Balance of space reflects a balance of life.

Even as the contents of our space can impact our psyche, they also reflect what is already occurring in our emotional space. If you have too many clothes in your closet, learning about the deeper reason for your accumulation behaviors can help you ameliorate them. If this chapter caught your eye, you may be one of the millions who hold on to unnecessary clothes and, though not in need of a true clinical intervention, would benefit from some assistance.

Why We Keep Stuff

Typically, we keep too much stuff for the following reasons: we think we may need it in the future; we cannot decide what to do with it; it expresses an internal state; it gives us a sense of security; or it has nostalgic value for us.

1. It is difficult to give away something that you might need one day. Lord knows you may need to listen to your cassette tapes one day when they miraculously trump our iTunes. That dead plant may one day grow some leaves. The screw you found in the basement may find the hole to which it belongs—right? Wrong! For most items, if you don't need it within a year's time, you probably won't need it at all. And if you haven't fixed a broken item in over a year, let's face it . . . you probably aren't going to.

2. You can't decide. There are two main reasons for the avoidance behaviors associated with clutter: you are unable to decide what to do with the stuff and end up doing nothing, or it is too difficult to confront the emotional pain that has led to the clutter.

If you don't have an organized system for stuff placement, clutter can add up. You don't know where to put it. Even if you have finally found a place for everything, you may find it impossible to address the question of what to do with the stuff. Both the *where* and the *what* must be decided before you bring anything into your home, but that is an incredibly difficult task for many people.

3. Your stuff expresses your internal state. A home that is crammed, cluttered, disorganized, and out of control may be an external expression of an internal experience, whether a past trauma or a current difficulty. If you are dealing with a job loss, the death of a loved one, a broken heart, or illness, why the heck would you want to deal with your closet? Avoiding the cleanup is part of maintaining your sanity. In these circumstances, it makes perfect sense to have clothing thrown around your home, piled in boxes, and still hanging in your closet with the tags. Eventually, however, the cleaning of the home can aid in the cleaning of the spirit. Have you ever seen a messy spa or retreat center? Would you want to relax in a cluttered spa or go on retreat in a pile of junk? That's what I thought you would say.

4. Clutter has its benefits. Being surrounded by our stuff is like having a life raft in a great ocean of nothingness. Our stuff becomes our security blanket that we have formed a faulty attachment to. Linus of Charles Schulz's *Peanuts* comic strip never went anywhere without his blanket, to the point that it became part of his identity. Is an avalanche of belongings in your home part of your identity? Do you feel less alone on a Saturday night when you have a pile of shoes on your floor? Are you less scared of the future with a plethora of CDs on your shelves? Do you manage your fear of financial ruin by storing enough food, paper products, and do-dads to support a small village?

5. *Your stuff reminds you of the good times.* I have saved the best reason for last because it is the most common and the most powerful. N-O-S-T-A-L-G-I-A! If I had a dollar for every time someone refused to give away or throw away an item for this reason, I would be a very wealthy woman. Your first tooth, a lock of hair, a baby shoe, artwork, an appendix in a jar—this type of item need not occupy every corner of your home. Even your brain undergoes neural pruning to eliminate the unnecessary; not every memory makes it. Use your brain and get rid of all that old stuff in your house.

Clutter, Closets, and Clothing

Clothing clutter is typically the least of the problems in a crammed home, and it can be one of the fastest and most satisfying areas to clean. When I enter a client's home, more often than not I find that she is saving her clothing for either the life she might have one day or the life she used to have. I hate seeing great clothes with the tags still on hiding alongside heaps of outdated or ill-fitting clothes in closets crammed full.

I usually see this type of behavior in people making a major life transition, such as weight loss, a change in relationship status, or a vocational shift. If you are going to go through the difficult process of losing weight, why not feel good about how you look while you're doing it? Wear the clothes that actually fit you *now!* Give away or return anything that doesn't work. Similarly, many women looking for Mr. Right keep the clothing they might need one day to wear when they are with him. News flash, ladies: you are not going to meet Mr. Right in your second-best clothing. Wear the good stuff *now!* Are you like some of the women I see who hate their cubicle job and dream of being in a more glamorous one? Like them, do you collect beautiful business attire that ends up crammed in the back of your closet in a godforsaken plastic bag? Wear the outfits. Who cares if you are the only one seeing them? You're worth it.

Another common reason for closet clutter is the deal-of-a-lifetime excuse. *It was so cheap, how could I get rid of it?* While I don't doubt that you can find some great pieces on sale that you actually need, the majority of sale purchases are impulsive and made only because they are on sale. In the long run, keeping those steals in your closet just because they were a bargain actually costs you time—trying to find a nice outfit amid the clutter—closet space, and extra money. If you don't wear your sale items, share the love and get rid of them. Use great sales to get what you need in your closet, upgrade classics, and add key trendy items to your wardrobe.

Sometimes when we hang on to clothes we don't wear and will never wear, we don't want to throw them away because we think it would be wasteful. But your efforts on behalf of the environment should not include keeping worn and stained clothes, accepting ill-fitting clothing as hand-me-downs, or wearing outdated styles. Giving away clothes you do not wear to those who can use them is a better way to eliminate waste and help mankind.

Some organizations take old clothing and blankets and recycle them for stuffing. Do your research to find those green-friendly places near you. Sometimes animal shelters request donations of fabric from clothing and bedding; there is nothing wasteful about keeping an orphaned animal happy and warm. If you don't want to see your clothing find a home too far away from your watchful eye, organize a clothing swap. Just make sure that the clothes you give or receive are in pristine condition, are current, and fit properly.

Clothing clutter is a great way to pad your life to absorb the jostling effects of fear—fear of not having enough, fear that you might need an item in the future, fear that you will have nothing to wear, fear that if you give it away you will give away part of yourself. Having racks and drawers full of clothing can feel good. It provides security in a world where often nothing goes as planned. However, when you are able to get past the fear and feel free to give away your clothing, you will find that your fear is imagined and easily conquered. It is in giving that you are freed from fear. Surrender, my friends.

Nostalgia is the nemesis of a clutter-free life. I battle nostalgia every time I clean out a closet. Can you look back on your life and remember what you were wearing when you got your first kiss? When you graduated, learned how to ice skate, or got your first job? These pieces bring you back to former times, but when you can't let go of them because of those attachments, you are a prisoner of your past. If you want to move forward, release the past, starting with your closet.

And finally, there is good old-fashioned avoidance. Opening the closet door can feel like entering the mouth of an undefeatable beast, one filled with clothes, shoes, and accessories. Sometimes it seems better to leave the doors closed in hopes that the clutter will go away on its own. You are stronger than this, my friend. Clean your freaking closet. Avoiding the problem will not make it go away, but mentally dividing your closet into more manageable pieces might do the trick. Start small and end big. If your avoidance goes beyond the physical space and into the emotional realm, you need to clean out the external *and* the internal places!

Are You Too Cluttered? A Checklist

☐ Are your closets and drawers filled to capacity?

☐ Do you have additional storage bins to accommodate your items?

☐ Do you have clothes and accessories in other areas of the house?

☐ Do you have clothes from five years ago? Ten years ago? Twenty years ago?

☐ Do you keep clothes that are stained and ripped?

☐ Do you keep clothes that are too big or too small on you?

☐ When was the last time you gave away an item in your closet?

☐ Do you have difficulty deciding what to throw away, what to give away, and what to keep?

☐ Do you find it hard to give away items because you might need them one day?

☐ Do you find it hard to give away items because you have memories associated with them?

☐ Does the clutter in closet cause you distress?

☐ Do you have clutter in other areas of your home?

☐ Have your friends and family suggestion you clean the clutter?

☐ Have they offered to help you?

☐ Do you avoid having guests in your home because of the clutter?

☐ Is dressing difficult because you can't sort through your stuff?

☐ Do you continue to buy clothing and accessories even though you have many?

☐ Does the thought of giving away your clothes cause extreme distress?

If you answered yes to many of these items, you are likely struggling with extreme clutter in your closet. It is time to examine what you have, why you keep it, and what you really need.

Case Study: How Unclogging Her Closet Freed Up Elle's Life

Elle was one such client who broke all of the clutter rules—in her house, in her closet, even on her person. It all started one summer weekend in Washington, DC, when she called me seeking clutter reformation.

"Hello, Dr. Baumgartner. I've been doing quite a lot of research on decluttering and organizing and found your information. I have been meaning to call you for quite some time, but I haven't gotten around to it. I really need to clear out some of this stuff as soon as possible because I am getting ready to change roommates. My old roomie cleared out, and people are coming by to see the place."

"Sure, Elle. We can certainly work on that. When would you like me to come by?"

"Well . . ."

Elle spoke at length about the process, the space, the time it would take, the amount of stuff she had, but when I attempted to schedule a date and time for an appointment, she would not commit. Eventually, I had to use a classic therapeutic technique on her: I gave Elle specific dates and times and asked her to choose one of them. This is very effective with someone who is indecisive and overwhelmed by the possibilities. Elle was trapped in her head, stuck chewing on the process. My very first task was to move her to action.

Picture a car going over the same path repeatedly; eventually a rut is worn into the ground. This rut makes it easier for the car to travel along the path, but also makes it more difficult to try another route. Additionally, the driver is led to believe that this is the only path to take. Perseverating about the process of clearing away her possessions was reinforcing a path in Elle's mind. Eventually, she became stuck, and her clothes were covering the alternative path.

After much prep time, Elle made a final decision to clean out her clogged life. My day with her began with falling over the items littering her porch. Before we even entered the closet, Elle wanted to discuss her progress thus far. She had read self-help books for internal examination, created a file to store any handouts, and bought a notebook to record the process and a calendar for goal setting.

Perfect. Elle was prepared. Unfortunately, when the time came for work, Elle kept procrastinating. Embarking on change is never easy. Beginning a task you've been avoiding cracks open the dam of pain, frustration, hurt, hopelessness, and anger and makes you face the unknown of the future.

Psychologist James O. Prochaska's transtheoretical theory divides change into six stages: (1) During the pre-contemplation stage, an individual is not considering change and does not believe that change is necessary. (2) In the contemplation stage, the individual examines the costs and benefits of change. (3) In the preparation stage (where Elle was stuck), an individual makes a plan of action. (4) During the action stage, the individual makes measurable behavioral change. (5) The maintenance stage is a continuation of the change behavior, and (6) the relapse stage is a temporary return to the original state.*

The true beginning occurs when action is taken. Elle was afraid to clean her apartment, so how was she to begin? In therapy with my clients or with family and friends, I have found that one of the least painful ways to initiate change is through the wardrobe. (The fashion

---

* J. O. Prochaska and W. F. Velicer, "Behavior Change: The Transtheoretical Model of Health and Behavior Change," *American Journal of Health Promotion* 12(1998): 38–48.

industry maximizes on this concept each season. Haven't we all fallen for the *It's a new year, time for a new you* line?) Changing what we wear is often an effective method for beginning a deeper change process. So that is where Elle and I started—in the closet.

"Elle, we aren't going to give away anything just yet," I assured her. "I just want to get a sense of who you are from your clothes. Let's begin by placing the contents of the armoire on the bed. I want you to tell me more about your pieces."

I made two important observations during Elle's wardrobe analysis. First, she frequently used temporal phrases such as "back in the day," "a couple of years ago," "when I was younger," "sometime in the near future," "one day," and "eventually." Second, she spoke about her past in extreme detail. I can barely remember what day it is, but this woman was sharing detailed memories from as far back as her childhood.

"My high school boyfriend bought me this when he went to Germany. It was around Christmas when he gave it to me. He said the sweater would keep me warm. We had such a great time just sitting by the fire together watching the snow."

Elle was stuck in between the life she'd had and the life she wanted, and her clothing reflected this state of limbo. Her clothes were either pieces she wore in her current life but found unsatisfying or unworn pieces (with tags still attached) for the life she wanted or the life she so desperately missed. Here was the starting point.

Finally, Elle, like the rest of her family, kept *all* of her clothes, and nowhere was this more evident than in her closet. Whether they were in style or out, fit or didn't fit, matched her life or worked against it, were old or new, were needed or unnecessary—Elle never got rid of anything. All these clothes were tightly packed into her closet like unfortunate sardines in a can.

The Golden Wardrobe Ratio

After seeing Elle's closet, I devised a closet treatment plan. To begin, we needed to eliminate at least two-thirds of her wardrobe. This is my *golden wardrobe ratio* for cleaning out a jam-packed closet: for every three items in the closet, two must go. No matter the closet, this rule of thumb has always served me well, even in my own closet. I usually know it's time to clean house when I feel that I'm not wearing as many of my clothes as I should or I'm having a difficult time deciding what to wear each day. When I'm done clearing out, without fail, I am left with merely one-third of what I had, my options have doubled, and the time it takes me to dress has been cut in half. (Yes, I was a high school math teacher in a former life.)

Uncovering the Past

Elle kept all of her clothing because she was sentimentally attached to each item. Every sweater, shoe, and pair of pants was a memorial to a special event or special person. Elle's closet was a living, breathing timeline of her life. Each piece documented her history, and her closet was the container for her story.

Cluttering behavior is often learned. Elle reported to me that, as a child, her home life was physically unstable. She never knew when her parents would have to move owing to unemployment, a new job, or a transfer. Holding on to objects as an adult provided her with an anchor to a family history that had always been in flux. She could form an attachment to something that would always be there. What was once a healthy coping behavior during difficult times, however, later became dysfunctional behavior.

Elle had difficulty parting with her clothes because she felt that to do so was to give away part of her history. She was an emotional hoarder of sorts—holding on to things because later, she might need the memories they evoked.

"I just feel so guilty parting with my things. It's like I am slowly chipping away at pieces of myself. If I don't have these reminders, where do I go?"

Learning to separate ourselves from our stuff runs completely counter to cultural understandings of identity in this country. We define the very essence of who we are by our trappings. When we give up our ties to our possessions, however, we begin to find out who we really are. The emptiness we try to fill by holding on to our things becomes filled when we are able to part with the very things we think we need. Many spiritual and religious practices include learning to part with possessions as a way to find spiritual enlightenment. Although cleaning out a cluttered drawer or closet may seem frivolous, doesn't this kind of activity make you feel better about yourself? Does it not also help you to question a possible purchase the next time you go shopping?

Elle needed to realize that her identity, which included her memories, experiences, and history, did not reside in her objects. All these aspects of her identity were already residing in every fiber of who she was. Because Elle's development had been shaped by her environment, she herself embodied all of her memories and experiences.

One of the treatments for clinical hoarding is to help people give away their items without feeling like they are losing necessary resources. For example, people who keep newspapers and journals are able to give them away once they learn that they can access such information on their computer. Elle was unable to give away her clothing until she realized that the memories attached to them could be accessed in her journals and pictures. She also realized that most of the pieces in her closet were unusable, that they were taking up precious space in her closet and her life, and that any memories evoked by clothing items that could not be transferred to other objects, such as pictures and notebooks, could be held in her stories and interactions with others who shared her history.

I took Elle to a large wardrobe mirror in her room.

"Look at the mirror, my friend. Do you want to see your history? Take a nice long look. Do you ever feel like you're losing yourself in your stuff? Return to the mirror. You are right there."

When Clothing Stands in for Goals and Dreams

In addition to the clothes that held memories, Elle's closet was filled with clothes that she "just might use," most with tags still attached. Long velvet formal dresses from high school, ballet leotards, Mardi Gras jewelry, lab coats—you name it, Elle had it tightly packed in her closet. She truly believed that one day an occasion might call for a Hawaiian grass skirt. Unfortunately, there are few luaus in DC.

I needed to convince her that her unused items were taking up room that could be filled with utilitarian clothing she wore not just "one day" but most if not all days. Purging her closet was a time to match her clothing needs to her current lifestyle and remove anything that did not fit in.

In her analysis, Elle realized that her clothes were more than just closet cloggers—they represented areas in her life that needed focus or closure. For example, it turned out that Elle kept that luau ensemble not because she might need it, but because she wanted to return to Hawaii one day to study the cuisine. Her workout T-shirts with tags still attached were still in her closet and not in the giveaway pile because one day Elle planned to continue practicing yoga. The never-worn "hot date" outfits had seen neither the light of day nor, more importantly, night. Between work, school, and too many dinners with too many frogs, Elle lacked both the time and the motivation to continue her search for her prince.

By removing unused and unworn clothing from her closets, Elle unearthed hobbies that had been lost but not forgotten, hidden dreams, and buried hopes. We often repress painful thoughts and memories in our unconscious, burying them far away from our awareness. Elle's closet represented her unconscious, a place where her unfulfilled and painful experiences, represented by clothes, were kept.

In therapy, specifically psychoanalysis, we must release the unconscious material and resolve the conflicts it creates for us. So too did Elle uncover her buried psychological material, identify the contents, and begin the difficult work of resolving the emotional conflict it had caused. Elle's conflict resolution began with signing up for yoga classes, setting up a vacation fund to visit the Big Island, and creating an online dating account with a picture of her wearing one of the many outfits she uncovered in the vast chasm she called her closet. As she slowly filled the six large giveaway bags, Elle began to reach closure with old relationships, long-gone friends, deceased family members, and times past. She realized that she did not need to hold on to her clothes in order to hold on to pieces of her life.

Your Turn

Is Freud in your closet too? Start emptying it, and you may find him!

You alone hold your memories and emotions. Objects become meaningful only when you attach emotion to them, but you can detach that emotion from your things if you choose to do so. Like Elle, you may be holding on to your clothes because they represent a significant event or person in your life. If this is the case, of course you would not want to remove any of these items from your closet—that would be like removing a piece of who you are! At the same time, sentimentality is the prime suspect in crimes of clutter. To keep your closet from becoming a shrine to your past, you can find other ways to document your memories.

When working with Elle, I noticed that she had hundreds of pictures to remind her of her experiences. These pictures were appropriate substitutes for her clothing. You might also find that pictures of events and people are just as effective as clothing in keeping your memories alive.

Another option is to take pictures of the items in your wardrobe; photos take up much less room than clothing. Some people may also choose to cut their clothing into small pieces and make a quilt with them. (If a quilt is going to become an unfinished project at the bottom of your closet, *do not* pick this option.) Use your imagination, but keep in mind that the purpose is to free yourself of the unused items in your closet.

When I think of anything in life that takes up mind space—like a cluttered closet—I always envision Marley's Ghost visiting Scrooge. He was weighed down by the very things he had worked so hard in life to acquire. And you? Are you being weighed down by the very things that are supposed to give you joy? As the Dalai Lama teaches, the road to tranquillity requires that we not become attached to our things.

Of course there are exceptions to every rule. There may be some items you simply cannot give away. Just don't let that be what you decide about *every* item. Try to keep your prized pieces in one container in your closet, your *treasure trove,* and do not allow yourself to use any more space than that container will hold. Feel free to decorate it with stickers, glitter, whatever. This is also an especially effective technique if you are trying to manage your children's clutter. If your treasure trove starts to overflow, it is time to consider which of the items must go.

You can use this declutter technique in other areas of your life as well, from schoolwork to social engagements, negative self-statements, and coupons. Life is simply better when it is kept simple.

If you have items in your closet whose purpose is to be available one day when you might need them . . . this might be the very day to let them go! After hearing enough declutter advice to last me a life-time, I can confirm that the sage advice of purging items you have not used in a year is relatively sound (with the exception of formal attire and accessories). If you are experiencing closet woes similar to Elle's, think about how well your clothes match your lifestyle. You may not need the maternity wear if you suspect that your pregnancy days are long past. My mother has a particularly lovely collection of new baby clothes and toys for her grandchildren, but considering that several of her children do not even have significant others, this collection is most likely extraneous and a *sublimated wish fulfillment* for her desire to have her now-grown babies back in the nest. Sorry, Mom!

If your clothes do not match your lifestyle, you may want to dig further to uncover the reasons why you keep these items. Are you holding on to certain clothes because one day you would like to take up tennis or become a tango dancer? Does that red dress—now a playground for dust bunnies—signify your burning desire to go on a date with a real man, if such a creature exists? Joking! Do you hold on to your size 4 jeans because after twenty years of inactivity and fast-food consumption you might, by some act of God and baby oil, fit into them? Perhaps the cashmere argyle sweater you wore many years ago on the day your boyfriend of five long years dumped you is crying out, "Move on!" (The sweater found a new home, and I . . . uh, she . . . found a new boyfriend.)

Just to give you fair warning, this uncovering, similar to the therapeutic process, may release overwhelming emotions that you are not prepared to handle. You may encounter feelings of loss, regret, self-disappointment, and hopelessness. These feelings are normal. Allow yourself to feel them, then embrace the opportunity to act on them and make positive changes. If you are keeping items because you might need them one day, consider this a signal that there are unresolved areas in your life and it's time for change. Listen to your clothes—they are talking to you. Your closet whispers.

Creating a Life Action Plan

If you are like Elle, you may need to create the life that you are saving your clothes for before you purge them. The clothes hanging right in front of you and overwhelming you can also create hope. Like Elle, you can consider letting go of the emotional ties to your past after you've created a plan for the life you want. This process lets you keep your memories within, not crammed under your bed in a bin. Internalizing your history will help you stop externalizing your memories.

Find a comfortable place in your home to sit and generate the life you have always wanted. To create this *life action plan,* choose three areas of your life—family, friends, hobbies, education, spirituality, significant others, vocation—to improve. Once you have chosen three areas, create clear goals for each of them. Then break down these goals into smaller, action-oriented tasks and ask yourself whether you can reasonably commit to completing these tasks every week. At the end of each week, you can assess which tasks worked and which didn't work, and you can add new tasks that will bring you closer to the goal. This action-oriented approach is perfect for people like Elle who are totally stuck in their own head space and never get their hands dirty to create real change.

When Elle began her life action plan, she chose three areas of improvement: vocational, interpersonal, and hobbies. For her vocational goal, Elle described a career centered on self-improvement, mindfulness, and personal health. She researched employment opportunities with health centers, alternative medicine, and spas in order to find her bliss. She also was interested in receiving extra training in health practices, so we found online programs, local centers for free informational seminars, and affordable training classes. Each week she was required to complete three tasks that propelled her toward her vocational goal, such as calling potential employers, sending out a résumé, taking a class, or developing a page on her new website.

The next area that needed some revamping was Elle's interpersonal life. She and I created the second half of her life action plan, the social calendar. As with her vocational plan, Elle was required to complete weekly tasks to move her toward her goals of having a more active social life and having a romantic partner. These tasks included crafting a profile on a dating website, asking a friend out to lunch, meeting locals at various events, going to happy hours, and inviting people over for dinner at her house.

The final phase of crafting Elle's life action plan covered her hobbies and interests, which included her love of food, flowers, and art. The beauty of these pursuits was that they were easily combined with her interpersonal tasks. Elle could go to a gourmet shop with a friend, see a gallery opening with her brother, or shop for flowers with a date. Elle agreed to combine these tasks to make her life easier and to pursue her hobby and interpersonal tasks weekly.

When the life action plan is complete, there is still more to do. You need the wardrobe to match. Examine each of the three areas you are trying to improve. Pull the clothes from your closet that are appropriate to the activities in these areas. For each weekly activity, prepare an outfit. If the outfit is missing anything, fill in the gap.

Based on her life action plan, Elle crafted other outfits for each event that she might attend, including interviews, social engagements, and events. Knowing how much she loved preparation, I had her write down each outfit and tape the piece of paper to the inside of her armoire.

During this process, Elle was even cutting the tags off the items that had stayed in her closet without being worn and putting clothes that were not "good enough" for the new life she had in mind in the back of the closet. I didn't have to say a word—her reassessment of what she wanted and what she had just happened organically. The life that Elle had always desired had begun . . . all she had to do was open her closet.

After you have completed the most exciting part of your wardrobe transformation, it is time to get rid of the clothes you no longer need. Purging clothes can create the most resistance in us, so complete this step after you have been reenergized by all of your life's possibilities. Once you're ready, the best way to examine how your closet became filled with unnecessary items and tackle the clutter is to use my Twenty Small Steps.

"Okay, Elle, it is time to get to the hard stuff—getting rid of the gunk clogging your emotional life, which seems to have deposited itself right here in your room. How did this closet constipation happen? And how do you want to clear it out?"

I left for the day to give Elle some time to think about the answers to these questions and to end on a high note about her new life and wardrobe plan.

Twenty Small Steps for
Cleaning Out Yourself and Your Closet

I have used the Twenty Small Steps with all of my clients with great success. The beauty of these steps is that you don't need a Dr. B there to help you with them. The Steps are user-friendly—you can do them on your own or with the help of a supportive friend or family member.

Try to get them done in no more than one to two days. Most clients require four hours of cleaning out and four hours of shopping, organizing, and restocking. Don't overthink this process—get rid of things as quickly as possible. Sometimes a Band-Aid just needs to be ripped off!

1. *Location:* Find a clean surface on which to put your clothes. The best place is usually the bed. If you can't find a clean surface in your cluttered home, find a friend or family member who is willing to let you borrow their space. The benefit of using someone else's space is the pressure you may feel to go through your items more quickly and efficiently.

2. *Empty:* After finding a space, take all of your clothing—and I mean *all* of it—out of your drawers, closets, bins, storage units, and boxes. For now, leave out your workout clothes, loungewear, pajamas, undergarments, socks, shoes, and accessories. We will get to those items later.

3. *Categorize:* In the clean space, separate your clothing into two categories: tops and bottoms. Tops include shirts, sweaters, coats, blazers, and dresses. Bottoms include pants, shorts, leggings, and jumpsuits.

4. *Focus:* After sorting your clothing into tops and bottoms on the clean space, pick a category. I usually like to start with the

smallest pile so as to improve the odds that the purge will be successful and to make it a little easier. The smallest pile is usually the bottoms.

5. *Placement:* Use large green trash bags or bins for throwaways and giveaways.

6. *Sort bottoms:* Immediately throw away any bottoms that are outdated, stained, or ripped. Give away any bottoms that do not fit you properly or are not the right length for you. Place the bottoms you decide to keep back in the bottoms section on your clean space, not back in your closet. You will go through them a second time after going through the tops.

7. *Sort tops:* As you did with the bottoms, throw away any tops that are ripped or stained. Too tight, too loose, or outdated? Toss it. Place the tops you keep in the tops section of your clean space for the second consideration.

8. *Assess:* Look at all of the tops and bottoms laid out before you. Do you have the basics, such as jeans and a white button-down? Do the tops and bottoms work together with their colors, fabrics, fit, and style? Ditch any item that doesn't fit in with the general theme of your wardrobe.

9. *Undercover:* Now that you have taken stock of your clothing, raid your underwear drawer for all of your socks, underwear, bras, and supportive garments. Throw away stained, ripped, or ill-fitting pieces. Anything you haven't worn can be given away.

10. *Function:* Do your underpinnings work with your clothing? If you have a ton of tube tops but no strapless bra, add that to your "to buy" list. If you wear tight pants and only have bunched granny undies, think about investing in thongs, seamless underwear, or boy shorts.

11. *Extras:* Next on the list are socks, night clothes, loungewear, and workout gear. Toss anything that is . . . well, you know the

drill. Give away the unworn, the never-to-be-worn, and the doesn't-work-with-the-rest-of-the-stuff pieces.

12. *Accessories:* Finally, tackle jewelry, scarves, hats, shoes, and other accessories. So that you can look at these items as part of the whole picture, lay them out with the clothes. Do they make sense with the garments that are now left? Do the colors flatter and work with everything you have? Are they quality pieces? Are they worn out or outdated?

13. *Look again:* At this point, your closet has been put through the first round of the Great Purge. Now it's time for a second look. Go through everything again. Repeat the process. If the second look-over is too difficult, take a day or two to walk away from the project and gain objectivity. Enlisting a stylish friend to help you with second-round decisions might be helpful.

14. *Outfit:* If you enjoyed paper dolls as a child, this step is for you. Have fun with the items you have left. Make some outfits, mix and match pieces, or call all of your friends over and have a fashion show. See if you can use what you have in a stylish way. Take notes on what works or take pictures of the outfits you love. You may find that yet another purge—number three—is hidden in this step.

15. *Reduce:* At this point, if you have done your job correctly, no more than half of your wardrobe should remain. When I am working with clients, my goal is to purge two-thirds of the contents of their closet. To date, I have always met this goal. Remember: de-cluttering should leave you with clothing that fits properly, has a flattering color palette, functions in your life, and makes you feel spectacular.

16. *Fill:* Have you looked through all of the items you have, given away what you don't need, and made what is left work? Okay, *now* you are allowed to shop for the missing pieces. I give you

permission to fill in the blanks with the perfect suit or just the right boot. But remember: each new item you buy from this point forward must replace *three* pieces from your closet that you gave away.

17. *Restock:* Make sure you have attractive containers and hangers for everything. Do not keep shoe boxes, plastic coverings, shopping bags, or boxes. Clutter be gone! Do not buy storage items for future use. If you don't want clutter to simply build up again, don't make room for it. Place like items together by season or category. I organize my clothes in order of warm-weather tops, warm-weather bottoms, cold-weather tops, and cold-weather bottoms. Shoes are classic brown, trendy brown, fancy brown, classic black, trendy black, fancy black, sandals, and formal dress shoes.

18. *Plan:* Put repairs in front of the closet. Find a reputable tailor and dry cleaner through family, friends, or local Internet reviews. Schedule a repair date and time.

19. *Enjoy:* Revel in your new and improved clutter-free closet.

20. *Maintain:* Upkeep is key to success!

Body Clutter

It's not just our homes and closets that can suffer from clutter and chaos. Your body can also be a clutter carryall. What my sister Gina has termed "body clutter" can come in many forms—such as wearing too much jewelry, accessories, and/or bags.

Jewelry

If you have ever watched Bravo TV's *Real Housewives* show, you have seen the finest examples of jewelry clutter our country has to offer.

MY STORY

Some people go on exotic getaways during their leisure time. Not me. I would take a good closet purge over a vacation anytime. The excitement of facing a great chasm of clutter, battling the beast, and surviving without being swallowed forever is unparalleled. The satisfaction of ending up with a wardrobe organized by color, fit, and function is delicious. The once-crammed space has been emptied and opened. Happiness is a clean closet!

One of the most fascinating discoveries during a good clean is realizing not only what you have but how little of it you use. If you have ever been privy to any organizational advice, you have heard of the *80/20 rule,* also known as the *Pareto principle:* for most events, 80 percent of the effects are from 20 percent of the cause. Applied to your closet, you actually wear 20 percent of what you own 80 percent of the time.

There are countless ways to test this theory. Some people hang their clothes the opposite direction after they wear them and later assess the percentage of clothes they have worn. Some people pick out the must-haves and wear only those for a month later, giving away the rest. I like to turn my clothes inside out after each wear and see what I've actually used at the end of the week.

There is no better way for me to gain a sense of control than to sort, throw away, and reorganize. The outcome, living with less, also provides serenity in the madness. Having fewer items to choose from produces limited choices and easier decisions. Additionally, because anything that is allowed to stay is considered a wardrobe "sure thing," I'm less likely to experience a fashion error and the terror of having "nothing to wear" is eliminated.

I recall a year I spent living in Newport Beach, California, when closet cleaning was of paramount importance. At the time

continues

> **MY STORY**   *continued*
>
> I was juggling graduate school and work, and my life was complete hell. Three-hour commutes at minimum into the desert, long days working with emotionally taxing cases, coming home to an empty apartment three thousand miles away from home, and spending free time writing my dissertation. One of the only cures for the emotional and physical drain of living like this was cleaning out and organizing. Cleaning my closet was a great way to create external peace amid an internal state of chaos. After a quiet night of removing, laying out, assessing, eliminating, and restocking, my wardrobe was cut in half. When my evening ended with a clear view of my perfectly folded, almost empty closet, I felt temporary relief from the daily frazzle, and the lightness of my stuff removed the weight of the day.

Diamond watches, earrings, bracelets, pendants, chains, rings, toe rings, and belly rings—all at the same time!

Why do some of us cover ourselves in more bling than a pirate plundering booty? Of course, we wear jewelry because we feel good wearing the sparkly stuff. For some of us, if one piece feels good, more feels better. Jewelry is fun, decadent, and totally unnecessary, which can seem to make it all the more necessary. Piling it on feels like devouring a chocolate cake whole—so bad it's good. Feelings of insecurity may be responsible when we wear lots of jewelry because we like to show it off. The more jewels we can display, the more successful, pampered, and glamorous we must be, right?

But often those who pile on the jewels may not know how to pick and choose what is right to wear for the outfit or occasion. Those who are uncertain tend to either go without or put everything on at once. Neither is acceptable for a stylish look. But jewelry can restore the pulse of a boring outfit if worn right. To wear jewelry properly, one must achieve *bauble balance*.

Balance with your clothes: If the jewelry is bold, keep the clothing simple. If the clothing is bold, keep the jewelry simple or don't wear it at all. For example, if your outfit already has decorations at the neckline, adding a layered necklace will look cluttered. A layered necklace is better suited for a simple sheath dress or a plain shirt.

Balance with other pieces of jewelry: If you are wearing a statement jewelry piece, keep the focus on that piece; there is no need to add more, especially in the same general area of your body. If you have chosen to wear huge chandelier earrings, forgo the necklace altogether. If you are stacking bangles, forget the lineup of cocktail rings.

Mix and match: If your jewelry is more subtle, you can wear more than one piece. But the days of buying a matching necklace, earring, and bracelet set are over. Be sure to mix and match your pieces for a more updated, youthful, and interesting look.

Accessories

Overaccessorizing is another plague on our style efforts. Kerchiefs, scarves, wraps, jangly belts, waist chains, sunglasses, headbands, hair ties, and shoes with hardware or detail can add up to a fashion disaster. When used properly, each of these pieces can enhance an outfit and the wearer. When piled on, accessories detract from the overall look and distract the eye. Accessories should complete your outfit, not compete with it.

So how to tackle accessory overload? Take my grammy's advice and "keep it simple, stupid." Less is more! Use your accessories sparingly. As with jewelry, try to limit yourself to *one* statement accent piece.

If you are using multiple accessories, choose no more than three pieces and make sure they are in balance with each other—such as an embellished shoe worn with a simple metallic belt and a pair of classic gold aviators. Try wearing one patterned piece with two plain pieces, or one bright piece with two neutral pieces. And if you are wearing jewelry, wear fewer other accessories, and vice versa. You can learn how to use accessories by observing the ads in magazines, watching fashion shows, and looking at your favorite designers' websites.

Handbags

Finally, we turn to bag clutter. Nothing is worse than a woman being bogged down with too many totes, duffels, and handbags or carrying what is clearly too much stuff in her bags. Now, you may genuinely have a lot that you need to carry around, such as baby gear or work files. If so, try to limit the number of items you take with you. Maybe you don't need your history book if you don't have that class until the evening. Maybe you don't need a whole package of diapers if you are only going out for dinner.

Most people don't actually need all the junk they lug around. Carrying around the candy wrappers, receipts, scarves, and so forth that can accumulate in a bag is simply easier than taking the time to look through the stuff. Frankly, this is a lame excuse! So pick a day each week to clean out your handbag and commit to it. (I always declutter on Sundays.) Dump out your purse or tote on a clean space and separate the necessary items from the stuff that just ends up there by default.

Sometimes stuff ends up in your bags because your home, closet, or car has reached capacity. Your bag becomes yet another container to catch the overflow of your life. Again . . . unacceptable. The bag is the easiest container to clean out. Take advantage of this chance to make one positive change in your life. Being successful at cleaning out your bag may trigger positive changes in other areas of your cluttered existence. Let it motivate you.

Consider what you actually extract from your bag on a daily basis: a wallet, a phone, keys, minimal makeup, a pen, a daily planner, work files, baby items. Anything else you don't use each day should be considered unnecessary clutter. Attack a purse or tote the way you would a cluttered home. Assessing what really deserves space and what should be removed will literally and figuratively lighten your load.

The "bag lady" look is not attractive. If you must carry more than one bag, limit yourself to two—such as a handbag and a tote bag—and make them attractive ones. Think leather satchels in soft, neutral colors or colorful canvas bags. Make some attempt at consistency. Your wallet, handbag, and tote do not have to match, but they shouldn't clash. Pick colors or types of fabric to tie the look together.

Finally, examine the dimensions of your body and the dimensions of your bag and make sure they are in proportion. A petite person looks ridiculous lugging a massive handbag. Similarly, a larger woman looks even larger if she's carrying a Lilliputian clutch.

Less Is More

Clothing, jewelry and accessories should enhance the self, not hide or distract from the self. Less is more, so choose a favorite piece and forgo the rest. The pieces do not have to all exactly match, but they should go together. The items can belong to the same color family (blues) or within a complimentary color family (black and white), and they can follow the same style (safari) or time period (art deco). If you are still confused about mixing and matching, watch TV, read fashion magazines, search style websites, or ask a friend. Focus on balancing the elements of your wardrobe—clothing, jewelry, accessories, bags— to make a cohesive and stylish whole. When people meet you, they should remember *you,* not your stuff!

~~

At the beginning of a long day or the end of a stressful afternoon, your closet should be a place of relaxation. When the inbox is full, the sink is filled with dishes, the dogs need to be walked and the children fed, the closet should be the one place that belongs totally to you. Let this not be the place that reminds you of the mess you need to clean, the clutter you need to clear out, the hobbies you don't have time to pursue, the weight you haven't lost, or the past you will not get back. This space should be the jewel box of your house, one that contains all of the wonderful items you use and love, that makes you feel beautiful and gives you the confidence to pursue the life you have always wanted.

A Note on Hoarding

Those who hoard often keep items that have no use, such as trash or junk, because they are unable to discard things. This excessive attachment to possessions creates a cluttered home and backyard. Those who hoard are unable to organize their possessions and they procrastinate in deciding what to do with them. In addition to hoarding behaviors, these individuals are often perfectionist about the fate of their clutter and limit their social interactions, owing to the mess. Hoarders collect items because they may need them one day, because the items have value, or because the items are emotionally significant. Often these objects increase the collector's feelings of safety.*

Hoarding behaviors usually begin in adolescence and progressively worsen. The initial symptoms include clutter and difficulty throwing things away, which eventually leads to a fully packed house in middle age. The root cause of hoarding has not been definitively determined. Currently, it is thought that hoarding behaviors may have a genetic component, since hoarders are more likely to have a family history of hoarding. Additionally, environmental causes such as stress, death, separation, or natural disaster may trigger hoarding behavior.**

Neurological research from the University of Iowa in 2004 revealed that the brain's prefrontal cortex manages the desire to obtain and keep stuff.*** When this area was damaged, subjects experienced an uncontrollable urge to collect objects and hoard them.

If you or someone you love is struggling with a hoarding disorder, help is available. Contact your local county crisis center (contact information is often found in the front of your local yellow pages) for resources that will help you clear the clutter, organize your space, and receive mental health care. Mental health services should include a therapeutic component, primarily cognitive behavioral therapy, and/or a psychiatric component for effective medications.

---

* Mayo Clinic, "Hoarding: Symptoms," http://www.mayoclinic.com/health/hoarding/DS00966/DSECTION=symptoms (last modified May 25, 2011).

** Mayo Clinic, "Hoarding: Risk Factors," http://www.mayoclinic.com/health/hoarding/DS00966/DSECTION=risk%2Dfactors (last modified May 25, 2011).

*** S. W. Anderson, H. Damasio, and A. R. Damasio, "A Neural Basis for Collecting Behavior in Humans," *Brain* 128(pt. 1, January 2005): 201–212; published online November 17, 2004.

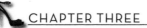

CHAPTER THREE

Somnambulist

When You Are Bored with Your Look

Finding the Pulse

Sleepwalkers are among us. If you don't believe me, take a walk downtown during rush hour. Check out the mall on a Saturday, or the metro during lunchtime. How many people can you count with a blank stare on their face?

There are times in our lives when nothing exciting happens. No major blips appear on the screen, and the Richter scale reads zero. Although it can be a welcome change from stress and strain to have nothing major going on, having all our days slowly melt into one without anything exciting to break them up is, well, depressing. Life is too short to navigate aimlessly—how many times have you asked at the end of the day, week, month, or year, "Where has the time gone?"

When your internal state is flatlining, your external appearance often follows. You twist your hair up in a ponytail or bun, brazenly displaying your roots. Your clothes are rumpled, worn, uninspired, monochromatic, or heavy on the neutrals. Finally, your shoes are worn-down, dirty, and completely practical. Accessories? What accessories? Does this sound familiar? A bland wardrobe is likely to reflect an internal feeling of blah.

You may have noticed that your gray, white, and black wardrobe is sucking the life out of your face. Maybe your safe pantsuit and white button-down shirt outfit is putting you to sleep. Are the khakis and polos decreasing your heart rate yet? Have your clothes become too safe, too boring, too mindless, or too effortless? Does everyone else around you dress the same way you do? If so, and if looking at them leaves you underwhelmed, it is time to shoot some adrenaline into the heart of your style.

You are not alone in this mild fashion error; many people in our country are suffering from this malady, a low-level kind of depression that I call *wardrobe dysthymia*. The best way to snap out of it is to take specific action to pull yourself out of the wardrobe funk.

Tired of Your Look? A Checklist

- ❏ Do you wear the same clothes every day?
- ❏ Does most of your wardrobe consist of multiples of the same type of item?
- ❏ Does your wardrobe consist of many basic pieces?
- ❏ Are your clothes generally unadorned?
- ❏ Are most of your pieces in neutral colors?
- ❏ Are your shoes in basic silhouettes and colors?
- ❏ Do you own few or no pieces of jewelry?
- ❏ When you go shopping, do you typically buy the same thing you already have?
- ❏ Is shopping a task rather than a creative endeavor?

❏ Do you buy clothes just so you have something to wear?

❏ Do you find fashion frivolous?

❏ Do you typically wear the same style of clothing no matter the occasion?

❏ Do you find dressing in the morning uninspiring?

❏ Are you less than thrilled when you have to dress for going out?

❏ Do you find that most people wear the same items that you do?

❏ Do you feel that you are just going through the motions?

❏ Do you find that most days just melt into the next?

❏ Do you feel that you have little that's exciting to look forward to?

❏ Would you like to make a change, but don't have the energy?

❏ Do you hope for a more exciting wardrobe, but just can't seem to make the change?

If you answered yes to a majority of these questions, both you and your wardrobe need to get a life! Once you learn how you got into this state and what you can do to make it better, some excitement is in store for both you and your clothes.

Case Study: How Sarah Finally Came to Life

Sarah was one of those people who had become apathetic about her wardrobe needs, but she would find the courage to make changes to infuse life into her closet and her existence. She came to my office stressed and depressed. She felt stuck in the decent-paying yet passionless job she'd had since graduating from college, she missed hanging out with her friends, and she had made "lose ten pounds" her New Year's resolution for at least three years running. It wasn't all bad—her relationship with her longtime boyfriend was going fine—but she felt that her entire existence consisted of making safe choices and thus avoiding the possibility of failure. She was tired of her life, not to mention her wardrobe.

"Dr. B, I am so sick of it. I look in the mirror, and what I see is so boring, so depressing. I feel like I have lost all the excitement in my clothes, but I am not quite sure how to fix the problem."

Our InsideOut appointment at Sarah's apartment was set for the next morning. I was eager to discern her reason for slowly allowing her wardrobe to disintegrate. Although this is a common dilemma, the issues at the root of it vary. Anything from perfectionism to depression can suffocate your style. The effect is cyclical: your wardrobe is blah, you look in the mirror and feel awful, you lose motivation to pretty yourself, and the wardrobe becomes even worse. Or you fall into the trap of thinking that if you can't put together a *Vogue*-worthy outfit, why bother (or risk) trying at all?

Upon entering Sarah's house, I was struck by the waves of tan and white in her surroundings. I saw no indication of personality, such as quirky knickknacks, a pop of color, or something old, slightly off, or creative. I was sure that this dullness would turn up in her closet as well.

Sure enough, behind the louvered doors was a collection of khakis, gray pants, black pants, black and white T-shirts, brown and black shoes, flip-flops, and brown and black belts. Now, I am a major supporter of wearing classic pieces, the structural components of a phenomenal wardrobe. But in Sarah's closet, where was the beautiful trim?

Like so many people, Sarah had a severe case of the clothing blues. What happened to dressing for dancing and Sunday brunches? What happened to beading, high heels, and wraps? What happened to glamour? What happened to Sarah?

"Sarah, what do you see here?"

"I see a super-boring wardrobe," she admitted.

"What would you like to see when you open your closet?"

"I would like to see something alive! Young and fresh. Definitely not this."

"Okay. Why has your wardrobe become like this?"

Sarah thought for a minute. "Well, I think that having these easy pieces, kind of no-brainers, makes for easier dressing. It's one less thing I need to think about, but now I am embarrassed that I definitely look like I put no thought or energy into my appearance at all."

"So are you telling me that you have this slight closet problem because you don't have the time or energy, or that you don't want to use time or energy to make an impact with your dress?"

"I'm just lazy. I want something easy, and frankly, what I have now is very easy."

"So why have you come to me now?"

Sarah went on to explain that when she went out with her friends, she always felt dowdy in comparison. At work, she realized, she literally matched the walls. Even on dates with her boyfriend, she felt that she was too predictable. Solving the wardrobe problem was going to be very easy. A couple of colorful tops and dresses, a sparkly necklace, a few hot shoes, and trendy belts would solve Sarah's problem. Unfortunately, there was probably more to Sarah's situation than just being bored with her clothes.

"So, Sarah, what kind of message is this giving to others?"

"I don't think it says anything. It is pretty blank."

"Do you feel that way, blank? Is that who you are?"

"Well . . . I definitely feel like I am going through the motions sometimes. I feel like nothing is particularly bad or needs major change . . . but I guess I could use a little jolt in my life."

"We can put a little spark in your wardrobe *and* your life," I told Sarah. "Let's get started."

The Psychology of a Rut

In a world that is unpredictable or stressful, many of us find comfort in a schedule or habit that, amid the chaos, provides us with an anchor. In mental health treatment, establishing a routine—for instance, by making a weekly plan—or having scheduled activities like daily moments for relaxation, a weekly date night, or a monthly trip is a very important part of patients' healing and return to normalcy.

The brain accommodates repeated behaviors. As an action is repeated, the neural pathway on which the brain signal moves becomes more easily traveled. Think of a wooded path that is initially covered in undergrowth, rocks, and leaves. The more you use that path, the more the debris is cleared, the dirt is exposed, and the dirt is packed, over time, to create a smooth surface for easy travel. Our repeated behaviors become easier to repeat because the brain signal travels more quickly.

Over time this brain signal no longer requires much effort, and if excitement and motivation disappear as a result, we find ourselves in a rut. Novelty is the answer to escaping from a rut. In 2006, Drs. Nixo Bunzeck and Emrah Duzel showed that the substantia nigra/ventral tegmental area, associated with the reward circuitry of the brain, is stimulated when presented with something new.* Additionally, the brain is hardwired to use novelty-motivation to seek rewards in the environment. Finally, learning in the context of novelty is enhanced. Novelty comes in many forms, and I intended to cure Sarah's wardrobe rut through closet novelty. Who knew that fashion is good for the brain!

---

* N. Bunzeck and E. Duzel, "Absolute Coding of Stimulus Novelty in the Human Substantia Nigra/VTA," *Neuron* 51(2006): 369–379.

Treatment

Sarah and I examined her life using her calendar as a guide. She had a full schedule of work, exercise, friends, and romance. There was nothing lacking accept change.

"Sarah, you have all the components of a full and wonderful life. It seems that you just need to add a few novel experiences to find some spark. What can stay and what should go?"

"Well, I really tend to like things status quo. I find comfort in my schedule. I enjoy doing the same thing, in the same place. When life around me is hectic, this predictability feels really nice."

"So what are some of your repeats?"

"Oh, I have many. I love this little Italian neighborhood restaurant and eat the same lobster ravioli every week. I love having my oatmeal and coffee every morning. I enjoy the same trail when I run, and I go to Fort Lauderdale to kick off every New Year."

"So you are a creature of habit and routine, but it seems that when those traits are expressed in your wardrobe, you are dissatisfied. Are you content with the routines in your life? Were you even aware of how much you have routines and repeated experiences?"

"Well, I always knew I liked the same thing, but describing it out loud is definitely eye-opening. To be quite honest, I can't think of a part of my life that is not routine. I think I would like a change, but keeping things as they are is certainly easier for me. As for the wardrobe, it is so concrete and literally in my face that I have no choice but to see it."

We discussed changes that Sarah could make to alter her routines while still finding comfort. We started small and took it from the beginning. In the morning she drank hazelnut coffee, so I had her pick out two other beverage options, such as tea or a fruit smoothie. She always ate oatmeal in the morning, so I had her add a veggie omelet and chocolate chip pancakes to her menu. She ran the same trail every afternoon, and now she had to pick two other trails and/or two other activities instead. Even the novelty of these minor changes would be good for Sarah's neuronal activity and boost her mood.

I returned to Sarah a week later to see how she was adjusting to these small changes. She said that at first she wanted to resist them, but eventually she realized that these novelties were exciting, and she actually looked forward to them. Adding something new to your life does not require moving to another city, finding a new job, or dumping your boyfriend—you can find joy in small changes.

I hoped that by learning the benefit of changes in her external world, Sarah would begin to see some change and growth in her internal world. Her ongoing assignment was to challenge her life with these new exciting experiences, each week pushing the envelope a little more. Maybe in a year I would learn that she had taken up cave diving in some remote area of the world, but for now we needed to turn to the reason she had contacted me in the first place—her dead wardrobe.

"Sarah, let's discuss these outfits you have been wearing for some time. Resistance to change is usually an indication of something deeper—perhaps fear of letting go, losing control, or making a mistake?"

"Hmm, well, actually I do fear making a mistake, so I wear what is safe."

"So, although wearing these boring pieces makes life much easier, the deeper issue is fear of making a fashion flub, which is nothing to be ashamed of. Many people dress safely because they really don't know how to craft a wardrobe."

Some people are born with this skill, and others are not. But those for whom crafting a wardrobe doesn't come naturally can still learn. It just takes a bit of guidance, practice, and a can-do attitude. I decided to take Sarah to the mall, where we could accomplish two major tasks: observing, through window shopping and learning through people watching. Although she had a fear of crafting and wearing riskier pieces, Sarah did have the ability to identify what she liked through observation. Once she identified what she liked, she could learn how to make the outfit for herself just by watching.

I based this exercise on Albert Bandura's *social learning theory*. Countering the theory that people learn solely through reinforcement, Bandura posited that people also learn by watching others, and he called this *observational learning, or modeling*.* Observational learning is a perfect way for someone who is afraid to make a fashion mistake to learn how it's done without suffering the anxiety.

"Okay, Sarah, we have arrived at the mall. Today I just want to take the time to discover what catches your eye. Once we have a sense of a look that you like, I can teach you how to make the same look in your own wardrobe."

Sarah and I sat in the main hub of the mall to maximize our people watching. A creature of habit, she was definitely attracted to simple pieces and monochromatic looks. But the looks she gravitated toward included a twist—one component that was oversized, outlandish, or incredibly avant-garde.

"I love this woman's outfit. The one with the black sheath and the thigh-high studded boots. Oh, this one is awesome, the white shirt, jeans, and diamonds. The girl with the pantsuit paired with the caplet."

"All right, Sarah, you like the simple with the pop!" I cheered. "Let's move on to the stores."

---

* A. Bandura, *Social Learning Theory* (Englewood Cliffs, NJ: Prentice-Hall, 1977).

We picked through boutiques, department stores, and bargain basements. Sarah was still stuck with a simple neutral palate, but she shocked it by choosing items that were completely full of life.

"Sarah, why haven't you done this to your wardrobe?"

"I have no problem telling you what I like," she said. "I just can't put the items together and feel like I stand out wearing them. I don't want to draw too much attention to myself."

Reidentification

Sarah and I spent the day crafting outfits. Since many of her clothes were already staples, I focused on buying the specialty pieces that captured her heart. I also showed her how to find classics with a twist.

We added:	We removed:
Multi-chain necklace	Thin box chain
Gold glitter heel	Beige flat
Tartan wrap	Cream pashmina
Leather motorcycle jacket	Black fleece
Pleated cuff shirt	White button-down
Longer, tighter skirt with a flared back	Black A-line skirt

Soon Sarah was ready to feel comfortable in her new skin. She needed to gain confidence in her style choices and adjust to the repercussions of becoming stylish . . . that is, getting noticed. In her new outfits, Sarah would receive attention from others, and she needed to feel comfortable with that experience in order to continue dressing that way. Although she had spent most of her life trying to blend in, she was willing to make a change and enjoy the outcome.

After a brief metro ride into the city, Sarah was ready to walk the streets of the nation's capital, during rush hour. To decrease her anxiety in her new look in the future, she would try her most daring pieces now in the thick of the crowd. If she could handle making a "mistake" or standing out here, she could handle making an error anywhere.

"Sarah, your desire to never make a mistake, to always look perfect, has led to a lifeless, bloodless, passionless wardrobe," I reminded her. "Where is the fun in that? This is a perfect opportunity to actually wear pieces that you love. So what if you screw up or get some odd stares? So what if you have a wardrobe mishap or someone laughs?"

"You're right. If you don't fall on your face a couple of times, you never learn how to walk!"

"Exactly."

Sarah was right where she needed to be—in the learning stages of crafting a fashionable wardrobe. She reminded me of the girl who puts her toe in the water before getting in, or the boy who insists on keeping the training wheels on his bike. Just like a good parent, I needed to encourage growth in Sarah, shake things up a little, and wake her. The time had come for her to stop playing it safe and try something new.

I gave Sarah a month from our last visit to try out the minor life changes and wardrobe tweaks I suggested. I was excited to see whether these small changes had infused her life with some spark and prompted riskier changes.

"Sarah, it's been a month. How is life for you?"

"So far so good. I have definitely learned a lot about myself. I realized that I was just existing, going through the motions. It took the wardrobe crisis to realize how mindless my life had become. Once I started making those minor changes, it pushed me out of a rut. True to form, I have actually included adding minor changes to my list of regularly scheduled activities."

"And the wardrobe?"

"Well, it feels good to take risks and creative liberties with my dress. Some days just doing something crazy with my outfit is exciting enough to make me feel alive the rest of the day."

There is nothing inherently bad about falling into a routine or a safety zone—everyone does it, and in fact we find great comfort in routines. But when these periods of arrested development last too long, stagnancy, boredom, and even mild depression may set in. When Sarah eventually acknowledged the lapse in her growth, she found the discipline and courage to make changes.

As I have always said, having a life worth living takes action—life doesn't just happen to you. You happen to it. I draw a parallel to being submerged in the ocean. Do the waves wash over you and pull you under? Do you fight against them until they exhaust you? Or do you allow the waves to help you get to where you want to go?

Your Turn

Finding Yourself

When you wear boring clothes, you are hiding from others—and ultimately from yourself. After all, clothing is the ultimate disguise. Put on a pointy black hat, black dress, black-and-white-striped stockings, and pointy black shoes, and people get the message that you're a witch. Your witch outfit sends the message to observers that, since you are dressed as a witch, you must be a witch and you must have all of the qualities of a witch. We all take mental shortcuts by finding the fastest explanation for what we see. And one of the easiest explanations of all is congruence: if the outside appears a certain way, the inside must match.

Call to mind a recent cultural phenomenon. As Susan Boyle stood onstage ready to perform on the show *Britain's Got Talent,* her look was not exactly aesthetically pleasing. Frizzy short hair, thick dark eyebrows, and a pale frumpy lace dress are not the characteristics we associate with a successful performer. When we looked at this woman, we expected an epic fail. We expected her talent to match her ensemble. We expected congruence. But when Susan Boyle opened her mouth, a beautiful voice emerged. People were shocked. How could an incredible voice come out of this package?

Sarah had been using to her own advantage our tendency to take cognitive shortcuts by making certain assumptions. If she wore clothes that faded into the woodwork, people wouldn't look too closely at her, both inside and out. If she played it safe with her wardrobe, others would not be on the lookout for her internal imperfections.

If you are using your clothing to cover a flaw or distract attention, consider addressing the underlying issue and treating it. If you are using your clothing to enhance what you already have, continue to do so. In fact, use what I call the *congruence technique* to your advantage: if your clothing is spectacular, most people will assume you are spectacular!

Finding Yourself in Another

We've all been there: we look around at all the exciting and stylish people, and then we catch a glimpse of ourselves. I had that "what has happened to me?" moment in Bergdorf Goodman in New York City. I know, scary, right? Wearing my usual NYC uniform of sneakers, spandex, and a long-sleeve T-shirt, I looked around to see all the well-dressed people. Those who took care of themselves served as mirrors pointing out my total loss of the self-preservation instinct.

Oh, I thought, *this is not good.* I had two choices: to stay compla-
cent in my bad choices or do something about them. As I walked
down Fifth Avenue in my scrubby duds, the ultimate walk of shame,
I took note of super-stylish women—many of them mothers, I might
add—who were wearing fantastic yet comfortable clothing. By the
time I entered the grounds of the apartment complex, I had devised
a plan of action to "kick it up a notch." Being stuck in a rut was not
the place where I wanted to be.

When we are unsure of who we are, or bored with the person we
have become, finding someone to help us find our way back to a better version of ourselves is often the easiest way to recover our sense
of self. Walking down the street, I could see my lack of self-care
magnified by the sight of those who took great care of themselves
and their appearance. Looking at them, I could finally see myself.

Grabbing my cell and wallet, I headed to the stores to find clothing that was both affordable and stylish, using my field research as a
guide. In no time, my sneakers were replaced by comfortable es-
padrilles, the workout clothes had given way to a spring dress, and I
was carrying a small straw clutch instead of my plastic grocery bag
accessory. The next morning as I headed back up Fifth Avenue, I felt
that my style revamp was well worth the humiliating revelation I had
experienced the day before.

My second *what has happened to me?* moment occurred on a post-
Christmas trip to Miami. The bright, beautiful colors worn by the
women in Miami—peacock green, flamingo pink, ocean blue—made
me take a hard look at my neutral wardrobe. A trip to a local mall so-
lidified my desire for color. BCBG was filled with colorful tie-dye, and
even Ann Taylor was swathed in navy, white, and coral. I was surrounded by female shoppers sporting colors, flashy accessories, and
sexy silhouettes, and here I was in oversized khaki shorts and a loose

white button-down. I had found my buried self among the women strutting down the cool, white tiled floor of the mall runway.

I have never been a bright color person, but my neutrals were neutralizing the life out of me. I started small, incorporating dark colors with brights. Naturally, being in Miami, I initiated my color infusion with beachwear. I traded in my boring bikini for an olive green and crisp white striped two-piece, my new cover-up featured an olive paisley print and beads, and I bought sandals studded with small gold ornaments. Even my toes got into the act when I painted them with a bright coral polish. After these alterations, my wardrobe wasn't the only thing that became colorful.

Look at the world around you to find inspiration. Is there someone whose style choices you find particularly attractive? Is there a woman you would love to hate because she always looks so put together? Don't fight her, join her. Through my brief acting experiences I have learned that we always have an element of a character we play inside of ourselves. I have played everything from a scheming witch to a prudish princess, and to play these roles I found the elements internally that I could connect with these characters and then amplified them.

You can do the same thing with your external self. Find a style role model, identify what it is you like about her, then identify those qualities deep inside yourself and foster them. When you are afraid to make those exciting changes, you can learn from her and then try it for yourself. You already have all the components of the internal self you seek . . . now make an attempt to look that way.

Self-Stagnation

Movement is good, stagnation is bad. Just think about the swarms of mosquitoes and accumulations of algae in pond water. When you are looking after a home, raising children, going to school, or managing a career, falling into a style rut is most likely a welcome change from the unpredictable life you may be experiencing. If you have had the same lifestyle for a significant period of time, your idea of "comfortable" may no longer include making the extra effort to wear the new and improved outfit. Without children or a romantic partner or career challenges, stagnation of the self is highly possible. Who hasn't gotten bored with their life?

I have spent the majority of this chapter stressing the maintenance of the self, but that self should also stretch and shift. If your environment doesn't require this of you, you must actively work to stimulate such changes. One of the most noticeable elements of the self that can get stuck is your external self—the image you choose to present to the world.

If you want to add spice to your life, make small changes first, starting with your wardrobe. Add one item that is a little risky. For me it was a bright color. For you it might be fishnet stockings. These small changes will lead to larger changes. These new items will more than likely invite compliments, which may lead to unlikely conversations, which may lead to exciting invitations, which may lead to a career change, and so on and so forth!

Extend this reassessment from your wardrobe to your life. I am a lover of routine and predictability, aka a control freak, but sometimes I have to stir things up a bit. What fun is a surprise party if you know you're having one? What fun is a blind date if you know the guy? What fun is a note from a secret admirer if you know who sent it to you? What fun is a mystery if it is already solved? Keep life exciting. If change scares you, find a guidebook, map, partner, or model you can follow. When you take the plunge into change, these items will serve as the lighthouse illuminating your way.

Madonna's career has been punctuated by change, and she is the maven of reinvention—the dominatrix, the geisha girl, the cowgirl, and even the born-again virgin! Most of us are never going to go to her extremes, but Madonna is an excellent model for moving forward. If you are wearing the same type of outfits over and over again, make a change. If you feel like you are blending into the walls, make a change. If you are tired of looking into the mirror, make a change. Change keeps the mind busy, the heart full, and the spirit young. Change is good.

Quick Tips for Reviving Your Wardrobe

Are you totally bored with your wardrobe but don't know how to build a new one? Are you afraid of making a fashion mistake? Here's how to instantly add life to otherwise basic ensembles.

Think contrast: For a sure way to make an elegant outfit, think contrast. Use monochromatic pieces in neutral colors with an eye-catching accessory that stands out against the simple backdrop. Think an all-black outfit with a thin gold belt and gold strappy shoes . . . a cream turtleneck and wool pants with a chocolate brown cashmere coat . . . navy pinstripe pants and a navy button-down with a light caramel belt and shoes.

Complementary and seasonal colors: Choose three of your favorite neutral colors, then choose one or two seasonal accent colors. Then all your colors will complement each other, dressing and packing will be easy, and the accent colors can change with the times. For example, choose white, cream, and tan as your neutral shades. Accent with aubergine and loden green for the fall/winter and with acid green and robin's egg blue for the spring/summer.

The statement piece: Dress simply, but pick one statement piece for each outfit. This is a piece that is colorful, sparkly, or artistic, goes against the norm, or is just completely different from what we are used to seeing. Consider a white summer dress with a concha belt . . . jeans and a pink button-down with a huge multi-strand turquoise necklace . . . white shorts with simple silver hoops and sandals and a wild paisley print silk top.

Trendy clothing: Don't waste your money on trendy clothing. Update your style with trendy accessories, such as shoes, costume jewelry, and belts. Your bank account and future wardrobe will thank you!

Designer brands: Find a designer brand you can rely on for style and fit. Nothing is better than knowing you will always find something that you like and that looks good on you when you enter a store or online site. These no-fail relationships can get you through the toughest fashion ruts. Choose a salesperson or wardrobe consultant from this store whom you trust. Often this individual will call you when new shipments come in, alert you about sales and email coupons, tell you about special services, and even find clothes that will work with your already spectacular wardrobe!

Re-create a look: It has never been easier to get the look for less. Choose designer outfits you love but cannot afford and find them at a lower price point. I cannot tell you how many items I have in my closet that people mistake for upscale pieces. I just look through the magazines and runway shows online, go to the cheapo stores, and re-create the looks. Seek and you shall find!

Internet resources: The Internet is your friend. Many of the major auction websites and classified websites offer clothing, jewelry, shoes,

and accessories gently used or completely new for a fraction of the retail cost. These sites also ensure authenticity. When I buy online, I
usually stick to items that have a registration number. If an item has a
registration number, you can take it to a store to authenticate. Before
I buy an item online, I email the seller, let him or her know that I am
going to take it to a main store for authentication, and ask if I can
make a return if the item is not authentic. The seller says, "Of course
you can return it." I save the email and have proof of the agreement.
These sites are not just for buying. If you are having difficulty ridding
your closet of unused or unloved items because you can't afford to replace them, sell them! Don't like the Internet? Then have a clothing
swap, find consignment stores, and even look through the racks at
thrift stores. Great gems are often waiting to be discovered.

Dress themes: Pick classic dress themes you like and stick with
them when you shop. (Notice I did not say "costume"!) Your theme
can be seasonal, such as French gamine for the spring, nautical for
the summer, English countryman for the fall, and snow bunny for
the winter. This is easier than you may think. Every year the major
fashion publications announce the trends for each season. No matter the year, every spring/summer includes a nautical look, a bo-
hemian look, and a black-and-white look. No matter the year, every
fall/winter includes an edgy leather look, a winter white look, a snow
lodge look, and a highlands tweed look. And every season I laugh at
how those "trends" are exactly the same as before! This summer I did
the safari look, which includes wide-leg linen pants, a fitted short-
sleeve jacket with wooden buttons, strappy sandals, and a wristful of
wooden or ivory and ebony bangles. I also did the exotic theme: large
lakh enamel earrings, silk print dresses, and low thong sandals.
Dressing and packing with these signature looks is incredibly easy
and gives you time to take part in the season.

Wardrobe repeaters: Spend your money on the *wardrobe repeaters.* You know what they are. The items you always wear, always buy, and always feel good in. These items are different for everyone . . . a string of pearls, a cheetah print stiletto, a pair of cowboy boots, a tweed jacket. I know that I consistently reach for jeans, a white button-down, cream sweaters, and caramel leather accessories. If you haven't found your wardrobe repeater, look to your style file as a guide. I noticed that I always cut out pictures of dresses with a built-in necklace embellishment. When I finally had the chance to wear a formal dress, guess what I bought!

Support for your lifestyle: I am a big supporter of a wardrobe that supports a lifestyle. Why would I collect clubbing clothes when I prefer to have a great meal at a local restaurant, walk on the beach, and drink coffee at a bookstore? Yes, I am unapologetically boring! Clothing should seamlessly fit into your current lifestyle, but it can also serve as a great motivator to go after the lifestyle you desire. If you would love to dance the tango one day, buy the clothes to dance the tango. Then, because you have agreed to my "clothing must match your lifestyle" rule, you have *no* choice but to use your tango clothes for the tango! This is my version of reverse psychology. You can dress for the lifestyle you have now, but why not dress for the lifestyle you want and go out and get it?

The downgrade method: When you are taking stock of your wardrobe, use my *downgrade method.* Visualize the clothing in your closet in a hierarchy: bumming around workout clothes are on the bottom, and black-tie formal wear is on the top. When you rid your wardrobe of unnecessary items, take everything you own down one tier. Workout clothes most likely will be pitched, and your casual weekend wear will now fill the workout wear slot. As you downgrade all your items, fill the empty slots with new clothes. Obviously, some items will stay in their slots, but the majority should be downgraded. This method will ward off the "I give up" look and keep you looking your best, even if you are only going to the grocery store.

The multi-function wardrobe: Create a *multi-function wardrobe.* Each piece should work across seasons and occasions. Before each purchase, I always ask myself whether the item is seasonless and how many places I can wear it. This method has saved me so much time and money, and you cannot even begin to imagine how it has changed the life of my wardrobe. For example, I wanted to buy a khaki three-quarter-sleeve shirt this spring. This piece was great for spring but could also work for summer, fall, and winter. The color and style worked with my other clothes. I could dress it down with white jeans and sandals or dress it up with a gold necklace, nude patent stilettos, and a printed skirt. I could wear it alone, under a leather jacket, or over a white tank. The possibilities were endless. Purchase made!

Get rid of it! I know you have heard this one before, but I need to say it again. If you do not *love* a clothing piece, throw it away, give it away, or don't buy it. If something does not *fit,* repeat steps above. If something is a horrible *color* for you, repeat steps above. If something does not fit into your *lifestyle* . . . you get the picture!

Falling into a routine is a normal part of life. Most of us enjoy the structure and predictability of knowing what will happen next. But the routine can quickly go from safe and comfortable to boring and depressing. You can find simple and wonderful ways to infuse life into the monotony of your day, such as drinking a new coffee flavor in the morning or using a new soap in the tub. Start simple. Start small. Start in your closet!

CHAPTER FOUR

Body of Work

When You Avoid Mirrors

I liken dressing well to wrapping a gift. When you give a present that you're excited about giving, you probably wrap it carefully in quality paper that has a nice weight, texture, and color and is well suited to the box. Then you accessorize the present with just the right bow or bauble. Before the recipient has even had time to open his gift, he has already assumed from the wrapping that a quality present is inside. Let your wrapping help you feel like an important gift.

Although others' response to you is important, there is no response more important than your own. When you look at yourself in the mirror, you must like what you see! There are many things women want to change about their appearance, whether it's a smaller nose, longer lashes, skinnier thighs, or bigger breasts. We convince ourselves that we're too tall, too short, too skinny, too big, or too bloated to dress the way we'd like. But short of surgical reconstruction, there is no better way to instantly alter your appearance and improve your mood than to dress well, and dressing well comes down to proper fit, proportion, color, and style. As you improve the way you look through your fashion choices, you begin to feel better about yourself and act accordingly—holding your head a bit higher, standing a bit straighter, and gliding through a crowd with ease.

If you are using clothing just to cover up your body, not only are you hiding your body, but you are hiding from yourself. Whether you are running from shame about being overweight, feeling excessively embarrassed about your post-pregnancy bump, or simply rejecting the body of the now, your inner demons will always find you. In this chapter, you'll find some ways to face the skeletons in your closet, and then revamp your look!

Appearance Anxiety: A Checklist

- ☐ Does the process of choosing an outfit and trying on clothes depress you?
- ☐ Do you avoid shopping because you can't find anything you like?
- ☐ Do you find that you avoid looking at yourself in mirrors?
- ☐ Are you engaging in unhealthy behaviors, such as calorie restriction or excessive exercise, to change your body?
- ☐ Do you see flaws in your body that no one else sees?
- ☐ Do you compare your body to others?
- ☐ When you compare your body to others, do you always feel worse?
- ☐ Does watching TV, reading magazines, or looking at websites make you feel worse about your body?
- ☐ Do you buy clothes based on the size tag, not the fit?
- ☐ Do you typically buy oversized items?
- ☐ Do you typically buy clothes in dark colors?
- ☐ Do you avoid activities because you are embarrassed by your body?

- ❏ Do you feel that as you gain weight you lose your sexuality?
- ❏ Do you wear clothes to conceal parts or all of your body?
- ❏ Do you buy supportive undergarments?
- ❏ If so, do you always wear them?
- ❏ Are you unable to allow your partner to see you undressed?
- ❏ Do you refuse to wear a bathing suit in public without a cover-up?
- ❏ Do you find that when you gain weight you lose self-esteem?
- ❏ Do you find that when you lose weight you feel better overall?
- ❏ Do you feel that people notice your body parts that you don't like?
- ❏ After you lose weight, do you hold on to the larger clothes, just in case you gain it back?
- ❏ After you gain weight, do you hold on to the smaller clothes because you hope one day to fit into them?
- ❏ Are you embarrassed to shop for clothing with friends and family?

If you have answered yes to most of these questions, you may have body concerns.

Whether you are just feeling the body blues or have serious body image issues, this chapter offers ways to find comfort in your clothing choices. If your feelings have become overwhelming or are impacting your daily functioning, you need to find a professional who can help you. Remember: you are not alone, and you can find peace. I have worked with many women and men who were struggling with body acceptance and who successfully achieved it.

Case Study: Why Clothes Loved Ricki Even When She Didn't

A week before Mother's Day, I received a distressed phone call from Amy, who was desperate to give her mother a much-needed makeover before their traditional Mother's Day brunch. Amy told me that her mom, Ricki, had a wonderful figure that was always hidden underneath baggy layers.

Amy thought her mother needed a stylist; what Ricki needed, I thought, was closet therapy. Most wardrobe mistakes have nothing to do with clothes but are almost always a symptom of a deeper issue. As I headed over to Ricki's, I was prepared to examine and treat her external issues, which meant cleaning out her closet and finding a better wardrobe. Only then could I examine what was inside.

When I met Ricki at the door, she was wearing an oversized, black flowy top and large black stretch pants that weren't exactly stretching—they were at least two sizes too big. No one would have ever known that underneath that blouse and hidden within the folds of Ricki's pants was a figure worthy of Marilyn Monroe. I couldn't wait to see the rest of her wardrobe and find out what Ricki was really trying to hide.

I began my wardrobe analysis by asking Ricki to clear a space in her room where we could empty the entire contents of her closet. I wanted to get her clothing out in the open so that she could begin to identify the patterns of her wardrobe mistakes. We sifted through the racks of oversized pieces and spread them out across her king-sized bed.

With all of her clothing laid out in front of her, I asked Ricki what she saw. She replied, "Lots of black stretchy fabrics and large pieces." Although that kind of clothing made up about 75 percent of her wardrobe, the rest of her closet contained clothes from the 1970s and '80s that were colorful, very fitted, and super-sexy. "What's with these clothes?" I asked. "Those clothes are staying," Ricki said. "They are from the good days!"

We split the clothing on the bed into two sections, tops and bottoms. Before even trying anything on, we trashed what was ripped, stained, duplicated, or painfully out of date (sparing Ricki's clothes that were from the "good days").

The next part of the process was for Ricki to try on each piece in her modern-day wardrobe. This is always a long and difficult process for clients: confronting the fashion mistakes they have been making to cover up emotional insecurities. Even more painful than identifying these insecurities is having to discard the clothes that hide them.

Every item that Ricki tried on was far too big for her body. I asked her if she thought that these clothes fit her. "Yes!" she said emphatically. She actually believed that she filled the spaces of her hanging waistbands, sagging back pockets, and flapping sleeves. I pointed to areas of bunching, puddling, and dragging on her clothing, a concrete way to prove to Ricki that her clothes were not for her body. The clothing did not fit the *now*. Ricki had a classic case of what I call *closet dysmorphia*. She chose clothes for the body she thought she had—that of a "big, ugly whale of a woman"—and not for the one she actually had.

Among the layers, baggy jeans, and oversized sweaters, Ricki needed to ask herself when and why she started covering up her body. Had it happened overnight? Had it always been there? Or did it happen slowly? Was covering up a response to a trauma or an inappropriate or unkind comment? Did she start doing it after her body changed in some way, such as a weight gain, weight loss, injury, or pregnancy? At what point in time did she turn away from the colorful prints, fitted silhouettes, and sexy styles of an earlier era?

"When did this happen to your closet, Ricki? When did you switch from these cute clothes to muumuus?" Ricki grabbed a deep scoop-neck dress with an empire waist off of her bed. The fitted bodice was covered with a knitted fabric, the waist was cinched with ribbon and a rhinestone buckle, and the skirt was composed of exquisite silk knife pleats. This was not only Ricki's oldest item, but her most loved. It looked like nothing else in her closet. She said she bought the dress in her early twenties during a time when she was "most happy" and "didn't worry about what others said."

Shaking the dress in her hand, Ricki told me, "There was a time when I loved to show off and felt proud of my body." But after she'd had her first child, she explained, her enjoyment of her body changed. Ricki then showed me a long, billowing teal top she wore as a new mother, the first of many oversized items she would collect in her closet. While grabbing her stomach, she said, "Childbirth will do that to you, but with this on, no one will have to see the bulge—not even me." Ricki tearfully explained that she wanted to show "a little skin" but her body wasn't "good enough" to do so.

Ricki needed to learn how to dress in a way that flattered her figure and boosted her confidence in her appearance.

Why We Hide

So why do we hate and hide our bodies? Unfortunately, we are often told to do so.

Ricki, like most women, learned from a very young age that her self-worth was inversely proportional to her body size—the bigger she was, the less she felt valued. During her twenties, Ricki felt that she was given a free pass to dress her body well because her body was worth dressing. In her words, "people could actually look at it *without* the cringe factor." But now that she'd gained a few pounds, Ricki believed that her body should not be displayed and wasn't valuable enough to wrap beautifully. As she told me in her closet, "No one wants to look at a fat lady like me."

As a natural part of getting older and having children, Ricki's silhouette had changed, but not as extremely as she feared. Her lack of awareness about the body she actually had was severe, and her fear of others' reactions to the body she thought she had was strong enough to compromise her fashion choices.

With such a strong societal emphasis on external appearance, it is not surprising that we internalize the need to achieve body perfection. Even though our model of perfection is false, often created with plastic surgery and airbrushing, we still attempt to achieve it. This self-induced pressure leads us to focus on and amplify our perceived flaws. When we receive messages that thin equals beauty, high value, and acceptance, anything deviating from the thin ideal induces shame.

Women like Ricki who believe that their body size does not fall in the category of what is deemed beautiful find their bodies unattractive. They make the further cognitive error of believing that if they find their bodies "disgusting," others must feel the same way. To hide their bodies and lessen the likelihood of negative judgments from others, they cover up with their clothing. They usually choose oversized clothes because they believe that loose clothes make their bodies look smaller, and they go for darker colors, which they have been told make their bodies look thinner.

Feelings of shame and loss of control over your body, however, can lead to unhealthy behaviors, such as starvation, purging, excessive exercise, isolation, and an inability to be objective in your perceptions of your body.

Body Image 101

The first part of treating Ricki's ailing wardrobe and psyche was to enroll her in my *Body Image 101* program. Together we would examine the root of societal images using retail and media experiences, challenge her faulty body beliefs, and learn how to assert healthy body beliefs. To examine and repair her poor body image, Ricki and I needed go no farther than her local shopping mall.

1. Lose the size tags. I began by taking Ricki to the mall and asking her to find a pair of pants that fit her at each of the five stores she visited. After hours of searching and much frustration, Ricki realized that the fit changed in every store. A size 10 in one store was a size 14 in another. So which pair did Ricki buy? The size 10. They were not the best fitting of all the pant options, but they had the smallest numerical value. When I asked Ricki to choose the store she would most likely frequent in the future, she said she liked the store with the size 10 pants and the store with the "skinny" mirror.

Ricki was succumbing to her own delusion: finding pants in a smaller size or a store with a skinny mirror was more important than the accuracy of the fit. So many women fall for these tricks! We promptly returned Ricki's purchase and found a pair of pants that fit beautifully. Before the new pants even made it into her closet, I instructed Ricki to cut off the size tag.

There are three things we all need to be aware of about sizing. First, clothing sizes are not standardized in the United States—just trying ordering from any online store with multiple designers. Click on each designer's sizing chart and notice the differences.

Second, sizes are inconsistent from one store to the next. If I can go to store A and fit into a size 0 or go to store B and fit into a size 10, I am going to frequent store A. Even at one clothing store, you may have noticed over the years that sizes that once fit you are now too big. This phenomenon is called *vanity sizing* or *sizing inflation*. Although nominal size remains the same, the actual measurements of the garment have increased. By playing directly into our obsession with maintaining the skinny ideal, vanity sizing makes perfect consumer targets of us all.

Third, the higher-end line of one designer is usually cut more tightly than the lower-end line of the same label. In 2003, Dr. Tammy Kinley conducted a study examining sizes and prices for women's pants.* The results showed that pricier brands have smaller sizes than cheaper ones of the same nominal value. For example, if you buy from Ralph Lauren, the size 2 in his lower-end "Lauren" line is far larger than the size 2 in his higher-end "Collection" line.

So why does this happen with our beloved brands? Maybe because the runway labels are more popular with European customers, so they run smaller? Maybe because, statistically, the women who have the money to buy clothing off the runway are thinner than women with less money? Maybe because this practice, by keeping larger women out of higher-end clothing, maintains the "thin equals beautiful" standards in the line? Vanity sizing isn't the only source of sizing questions. We could also ask why, if the average female is a size 14, the clothing we find in stores rarely goes beyond a size 10 or 12, leaving larger women no choice but to shop in "special" stores that do not include mainstream designers.

Although we may never have all the answers, asking critical questions will make you feel powerful enough to conquer, rather than consume, the fashion information in front of you.

2. *Filter your media.* Clothing stores aren't the only breeding grounds for poor body image. All we need to do is open a magazine or watch television to learn what we "should" look like. Well, we can't blame the media for everything, but the mentions and images of diets, weight loss, models, celebrities, and so forth that constantly bombard us are certainly convincing.

---

* T. R. Kinley, "Clothing Size Variation in Women's Pants," *Clothing and Textiles Research Journal* 21(1, 2003): 19–31.

I asked Ricki to watch TV for a week with the idea of identifying the direct or indirect messages she was receiving about female beauty. At the end of the week, I asked her what she had learned about what is considered most beautiful, and she responded, "Young and thin." I put Ricki on a strict media diet until she was able to fix the filter through which she viewed it. If she believed that her body was damaged from gaining weight, the content of magazines and television would simply confirm that belief. Only when she had changed her understanding of her body and begun to believe that she had value with or without a svelte exterior could she look at media without internalizing its often unhealthy message. She would then see these images and not feel that she should attempt to look like them. She would understand that media images are not only doctored but do not even represent the majority of the female population. For now, Ricki promised herself that if she saw a show or looked at an ad that made her feel horrible about her own body, she would change the channel or turn the page.

Fix your filter by examining media images with a critical eye. These images are not real. Detach yourself from the women you see; do not attempt to relate to them. If this is too difficult for you to do, then avoid contact with the images. This may mean turning off the television or temporarily canceling your subscriptions.

Once you have considered and come to understand all of the external factors that arbitrarily impact your body image and ultimately your fashion choices, turn toward the mirror. The person responsible for accepting and properly packaging you is you.

3. *Exposure therapy*. When we experience anxiety like Ricki's fears about her body, turning to an avoidance mechanism, such as hiding under baggy clothes, takes the anxiety away in the short term but strengthens it in the long term. The next part of my treatment required that Ricki take action to combat her body image anxiety rather

than avoid it. Through cognitive behavioral therapy (CBT)—which is based on the theory that faulty thoughts negatively impact emotions and behaviors—I set up experiments designed to challenge Ricki's beliefs, feelings, and past experiences related to covering up. So, in order to reduce her anxiety, Ricki had to confront it by takin' it all off, baby!

I took Ricki back to the mall on a busy Friday night. As we walked past the movie theater lobby packed with teens and their parents, I knew this would be the perfect place to make Ricki the most uncomfortable. If you can survive being stared at and possibly judged by a group of adolescent girls without crumbling, you can handle almost anything, I assured her.

Ricki stood in the lobby wearing a tank top I had borrowed from her daughter and an old pair of tight jeans from her "good days." She was in the thick of the *in vivo* experiment . . . and she wasn't happy. She felt exposed, embarrassed, vulnerable, and ugly. She felt that all of the moviegoers were staring at her, all of the laughter was directed at her, and all of the conversations centered on her "horrific body." After standing in the lobby, Ricki and I walked to the next busy location—the mall cafeteria.

What began as an exercise in merely surviving a worst-case scenario became an exercise in questioning current beliefs. Walking around the mall in a tank top turned out not to be as bad as Ricki had thought it would be; in fact, her outfit helped her keep cool in a packed mall. She also noticed that other women, many of whom she believed looked better than she did, covered their bodies. She also noticed that nobody noticed! Nobody was shocked by seeing Ricki in a tank top, no one cared that her arms were soft, and no one shrieked in horror at her semi-exposed body.

Ricki got through the worst part of the wardrobe therapeutic process: facing her fear of body exposure in front of others. Although

her body concerns were not going to dissipate after just one intervention, she could begin to see that there was an alternative way to look
at her body and alternative options for her wardrobe. She realized
that her fears of exposure were based more on her own faulty perceptions of her body than on the responses of others. She discovered
that the responses she thought she received were her own responses
projected onto others. In other words, *if I think my body is disgusting,
then surely others must think so too.* The only person stopping Ricki
from wearing sexy clothes was Ricki. She also learned from this experiment that attractive can come in all different sizes. She saw
many women in the mall who were larger than her but who were
wearing clothing she was too afraid to wear.

4. Deflection. The last part of the internal treatment was to teach
Ricki how to respond to negative feedback from others, such as
stares, sneers, eye rolls, and silent treatments that Ricki swore were
directed at her. If Ricki was going to make a style transformation, she
would need to risk possible criticism from those who were content
with her dressing patterns. I explained to Ricki that I am always
amazed by friends and family who, after begging for style help on behalf of their "loved ones," present the most resistance to change.

Ricki was coming to an important realization: "I have spent so
many years fearing what others might say about my body that I think
I've lost the ability to defend my own fashion choices!" So we worked
on assertiveness techniques—ways to let any potential critics know
that Ricki found their negative comments offensive. We began slowly
through role-play. I asked Ricki to list all of the possible criticisms
that others could hurl at her. *Fat, heifer, disgusting, slob,* and *hideous*
were a few of the awful taunts Ricki listed. After writing these down,
I sat across from her and, in the best mean girl voice I could muster,
called her every name on the list. Like anything you are exposed to

many times, the initial negative impact of the words decreased as I re-peated them.

I then asked Ricki to generate responses to these taunts that would maintain her sense of dignity and power. We used deflection techniques similar to the ones I use with difficult patients in therapy, phrases such as "I am sorry you feel that way," "That's an interesting comment," and "That's great that you have an opinion!" We also used direct confrontation phrases such as "You have a right to your opinion, but your comments are hurtful," and "I find your behavior inappropri-ate and am leaving this room if you are unable to change it." After choosing her favorite responses, Ricki felt prepared to confront a critic from a place of strength rather than emotional vulnerability.

We then immediately applied Ricki's deflection phrases. As when a patient in therapy learns a new skill, I do not wait to apply it. Skills applied immediately in the office are more likely to be remembered and to be applied elsewhere successfully. If Ricki was immediately confronted with the real situation, she would remember that she al-ready had the skill to successfully defend herself. So I said something horribly rude to Ricki: "Wow, you look really awful in those pants." Her reply? "Well, that's unfortunate that you think that way." Success! After many practice runs, Ricki's rehearsed responses became her de-fault stock phrases.

When you are caught off guard, having a go-to response or catch-phrase is essential because high emotions will interfere with your normal cognitions. If you can think now about the worst thing that someone could say about you, generate an effective response, and then *practice* this response with someone you trust, you will be pre-pared to implement this deflection technique in the real world.

As Ricki felt more comfortable with her assertiveness skills, we went out into "the field." She was prepared to confront anyone who criticized or shamed her. But to her happy surprise, as I predicted, the fieldwork failed miserably. The worst never came. As Ricki dressed and acted with only herself in mind, she had no room for the projected opinions of others. She finally realized that the opinion she had feared the most for so long might have actually been her own.

Reidentification

Ricki and I had a trying week as we looked through her closet, identified the internal roots of her wardrobe malfunctions, and confronted her inner demons, but she had grown emotionally stronger along the way. Now we were ready for the fun part: curating her style and restocking her empty closet.

"So, Ricki," I asked, "if you had the 'perfect' body, what would you wear?" She gathered the clothes from the "good days" into a neat pile. Aside from her favorite dress, I asked her to walk me through her three favorite pieces and tell me why she was attracted to them. I can often use components of clothing from an old wardrobe to guide new wardrobe decisions about color, fabric, or embellishment. (Using pictures of favorite styles is equally effective.)

Ricki pulled out a button-down shirt, fitted pants, and a long dress. When I asked her why she liked the sheer fitted silk button-down, she said that the aubergine color and the long tie at the collar made her feel "feminine and sophisticated." We looked next at the tuxedo pants. Ricki loved that the pants were multi-functional: she could go from work to a cocktail party wearing them. Finally, we turned to the column maxi-dress in hot pink. The dress "covered" her, Ricki said, but it also showed off her figure, and the color made her "stand out from the crowd."

After we discussed these favorite pieces and filled bags with clothes we had mutually rejected, I sat Ricki down on her couch and created a style wish list that she would use when shopping for her new wardrobe. We knew that she responded to clothes that made her feel sexy, feminine, and sophisticated. She also enjoyed soft and sheer fabrics like silk and cashmere in bright colors and prints.

To create a wardrobe that matched Ricki, I wanted to strip away everything extraneous, get down to the very essence of her, and then dress this essence. I sat with her in her room and asked her to tell me about herself as well as her body, to describe for me what she thought of her body regardless of how others responded to it, and to think about what message she wanted to convey to others. I gave Ricki pencil and paper and told her to get to work.

After spending some time scribbling and erasing, Ricki blurted out, "Darn it, I'm sick of fading into the background. I am not invisible. When I walk into a room, I want to leave a wake behind me."

Oh, here it is, I thought. *The good stuff.*

I asked her what a woman who feels that way about herself might wear. "She would wear sexy clothes while remaining a lady," Ricki responded. It was clear that Ricki wanted to feel young and fresh, but as a woman, not as a teenager. I probed further, asking her to imagine how a woman who is all those things would dress. "Color, prints, and sparkly jewelry," she said with clarity and conviction.

We shopped for the woman Ricki wanted to be and, in fact, always was before she began ignoring and covering her essence. We purchased items like Diane von Furstenberg wrap dresses in colorful prints. These dresses happened to be made in stretch fabrics that accentuated her bust, waist, and legs but camouflaged her tummy. Ricki also loved sexy and modest fitted turtlenecks—they reminded her of the sirens of film noir—and they happened to show off her figure without exposing her and making her feel vulnerable. Fitted and flared pants accentuated her femininity and also happened to maximize her greatest asset.

Ricki's new wardrobe didn't make her feel confident: her clothing was simply the physical representation of the emerging confidence she already felt. I explained to Ricki that, like any other emotion, confidence has its good days and its bad days. She might wake up one morning and feel that she could take on the world. On other days, she might wake up and want to crawl right back into bed. As in therapy, I helped Ricki create an emotional "emergency kit" for those bad days. She committed to doing at least one hour of exercise, making one phone call to reach out to a friend, and wearing one hot outfit. With her newfound confidence, spectacular wardrobe, and safety plan in place, Ricki felt ready to face the world—as Ricki.

Ricki and I spent the evening before her much-anticipated Mother's Day brunch unwrapping clothes and hanging them in her closet. These clothes, in Ricki's words, captured her inner strength and passion for life. For the brunch, Ricki chose a fitted and flared cream shantung silk suit with a pastel plaid silk shantung shell and nude stilettos. Her outfit was a hit. Amy, Ricki's daughter, felt that she had her mother back. "She was so unhappy for so long," Amy told me. "Her look finally matches the person she is on the inside. I knew my mom was in there somewhere . . . I'm just glad she finally came out!"

I am happy to report that Ricki's transformation was a permanent one. She still slips into the muumuu mode occasionally, but rather than declare defeat, she mobilizes her emergency coping strategies. She puts on her Richard Simmons workout tapes and wears her favorite outfit afterward. She still dreads shopping for clothes, but relishes choosing her outfits from her own closet. She told me recently that the "good days" are back.

Your Turn

Look at each piece of clothing in your closet as one component of your emotional timeline. When did you stop dressing for the body you actually have? When did you start using clothes to hide? When did you begin to wear dark colors to cover the flaws?

Try to remember when and why you bought each garment you own. Did you buy it because you were going out in public and wanted to remain enclosed? Did you buy it out of desperation because you felt that nothing else looked good on you? Let the fabrics of your closet weave the emotional history of the internal you. Try to identify the roots of your emotional landscape as evidenced in your wardrobe.

Keep in mind that thought without action can lead to paralysis of analysis. Simply looking at your closet will not move you toward change. As Ricki did with the exercise from cognitive behavioral therapy, you must take action. As a sample CBT experiment, remove one layer of clothing you are wearing, first by yourself, then in the presence of another. If you are wearing a cardigan over a sleeveless dress, remove the cardigan. But before you do, examine your anticipation of uncovering. Are you nervous? If so, why? How do you think you will feel? What might others think? How will you handle your discomfort?

After the experiment, examine your cognitive reactions. Were you uncomfortable? If so, why? What were your fears about others' reactions? What were their actual reactions? What did you feel about yourself? Was the anticipation worse than the actual experience? Where do these feelings come from? Childhood? Adolescence? Adulthood?

Each time you try this experiment and the ones that follow, you can push yourself a little further out of your comfort zone and learn to cope with the anxiety of the situation. As you work slowly through the emotional layers, you may notice yourself shedding external layers too. When you do, you will know that you're getting comfortable in your skin.

Act "As If"

Another technique I use in therapy is called *act as if*. Act as if you have a perfect body. Act as if you love your body. How would a person with body confidence behave? If you're confused about how to act as if you love your body, just go to the beach. Look at all of the men who proudly expose their beer bellies and all the women who comfortably play in the water, cellulite and all.

When you act "as if," you change your behavior, which facilitates positive changes in your thoughts and emotions. For example, if you act as if you have confidence in your body, you will choose the knock-out dress. Maybe you receive a compliment or two or simply catch a glimpse of yourself in the mirror and smile. Experiences like this may help you question your assumption that your body is unattractive and also help you feel happier about what you see, encouraging more confident clothing choices in the future.

If you have spent years torturing yourself about your body, changes will not occur overnight. Whether you are attempting to change through "act as if" or through closet analysis, you must first confess to the lie of hiding, covering, and camouflaging, or the deception of buying sizes that are too small for you or only caring for the skinny mirror.

All of us have times when we must reassess the shell that contains the person inside, and the process is uncomfortable. You will know that you need to reassess when dressing in the morning is not as pleasurable as it used to be, or when you are just not feeling as confident as you once did. When you feel that something in you is "off," it's time to figure out what's really going on.

Fear of Shopping: You Deserve to Dress Well

Some people view shopping and dressing as necessary chores. Those who do not like these tasks usually do not like how they look. Trying on clothes and looking at their reflection in the mirror provides further imagined evidence that they are not attractive. I know the feeling—when I feel horrible about myself, nothing is worse than trying on clothes, only to be horrified by what I see in the dressing room mirror. I have to fight the urge to go home, put on my robe, light a candle, and eat raw cookie dough.

What is even more often the case is that people do not like shopping and dressing because they don't know how to find clothes that are right for them and they don't know how to assemble outfits effectively. My sister Gina hated going shopping, and she hated picking out outfits to wear from her closet just as much. She often used the word "overwhelming" when describing her shopping excursions; in fact, she felt that shopping was a form of punishment. When she shopped, Gina had no clear idea of what she liked, what looked good on her, what she needed in her closet, where to find various items, and how to put it all together. When she tried to pick out clothes from her closet, she didn't know what she already had, what clothes went together, what fit her, when to give away an item, and when to revive an item.

To help Gina learn how to have a successful shopping experience, I had her identify the types of looks she liked, either by looking at pictures or by browsing in stores. Then we looked through her wardrobe to find pieces that matched the looks she loved, and we removed all those items that didn't work with her look. Finally, we went to the store to pick out pieces that worked with her identified look, fit her properly, matched her lifestyle, and made her feel better when she wore them.

I also helped her remove personal insults—"My body doesn't work with these clothes," "I look awful," "Nothing looks good on me"—from the process. After Gina adopted a non-emotional, objective approach, she saw that something either worked or it didn't. With this assistance, and through some trial and error, Gina learned to shop on her own and make the experience efficient, productive, and pleasurable!

Once you learn what you love and what looks good on you, dressing can only be a positive, if not an uplifting, experience. Just like eating a delicious meal or having a relaxing massage, putting on clothes that look and feel spectacular can only make you feel better.

Wearing your clothes engages all of the senses. You can be calmed by a muted beige wrap with shell adornments or brightened by an orange satin cocktail dress with magenta sandals. You can hear the tinkling of silver bangles or the *swoosh* of a party dress when you turn a corner. You can feel the soft faux fur pelt around your neck or melt into a pair of charmeuse pants. The next time you try on clothes from your closet or in a store, see if you can use this experience to gauge your senses. This can not only help you decide on the items you find most wonderful but turn your focus away from the perils of picking out clothes.

There is nothing worse than going to a store with friends or a client, seeing them try on something that looks spectacular on them and makes them love the way they feel, but then watching as they walk away because they "just can't." They are saying, "I just can't," not because they cannot afford the item, but because they feel uncomfortable spending their own hard-earned money on themselves. Those who say, "I just can't," are the ones who feel as though they need to justify every purchase to themselves or to others.

To everyone who's ever said, "I just can't," I would remind you that you never need to feel guilty—or let anyone else make you feel guilty—for taking the time, effort, and money to dress well and treat yourself well.

As I stated at the beginning of this chapter, anything that is worthwhile on the inside deserves a wonderful wrapping. So why don't you begin to wrap yourself well? I believe you should dress yourself in the best clothes that you can afford. When it comes to clothing, you usually get what you pay for, so why not get yourself something you love, even if it costs more?

The psychological concept of *exposure therapy* is relevant here. If you continuously expose yourself to something that makes you anxious while also practicing relaxation techniques, you can eventually learn to overcome your anxiety. Exposure therapy is usually used with people who have various phobias or suffer from panic attacks. Applied to shopping, this means that you can go ahead and experience all the anxiety and guilt you're used to feeling when buying nice things, but eventually, if you buy nice things in spite of your self-judgment or the judgment of others, you will reduce those feelings.

Sometimes we worry about what people will think of us when we wear something nice, or we fear the person in our social circle whose first remark is always about what we are wearing. I have known a couple of these amateur fashion critics (who are always the most poorly dressed people in the room) and heard their passive-aggressive comments, such as "What are you wearing?" "Oh, that outfit is . . . interesting?" They have neither a kind word to say nor a kind look. One of these "critics" would consistently ask me why I was "so dressed up" even when I was wearing jeans and a button-down! Notice that she never said that I "looked nice," just that I was "so dressed up." I used to dress for this kind of person, hoping to avoid the self-esteem-killing comments. But in doing so, I did the very thing I was trying to avoid—I was weakening my sense of identity and *decreasing* my self-esteem. Now I simply dress as I want to. I might even wear the very things that would really drive these people crazy!

Buying something wonderful for yourself is like any other form of pampering: it can often have positive long-term effects, especially if the item makes you feel spectacular every time you wear it. As we all know, you must first use the oxygen mask on the plane before you can put one on a child sitting next to you. Before you can take care of others, you must first take care of yourself.

One of the easiest ways to take care of yourself is to take the time to find flattering clothes and then actually wear them. Don't worry about how your old self would feel about taking care of yourself this way, stop waiting for the stars to align before you wear something nice, don't listen to whispers about how much you might have spent, and simply don't answer the question "Why are you so dressed up?" Dress well on the outside to help yourself glow from the inside.

Quick Tips for Making the Most of What You Have

Too tight: Shrink-wrapping yourself into your clothing will not fool anyone. You will not look a size smaller; in fact, you'll only make yourself look even larger. Keep casings for your sausages. If you see a pull, stretch, rip, or strain, do not buy or wear the item. Sizes are not standardized in the United States, so a size 2 may be a size 10 in another store, or even within a designer's other lines. Ignore the number. It does not measure your worth! Just find the right size.

Too loose: Would you put a sack over the *Mona Lisa*? Would you cover a garden of roses with a blanket? Then why in the world would you wrap yourself in an oversized garment? Do not hide from the world. Find outfits that fit you properly, which means fitting the largest part of your body and tailoring the rest if necessary. If you are confused about fit, do your research. Look on the Internet at fashion websites to examine fitting guidelines, enlist the help of a sales associate, or contact a reputable tailor. If it is comfort you seek, there are alternatives to the oversized sweatshirt or sagging yoga pants. Try a great wrap dress or jeans. Trust me, your audience will prefer it to your ratty ensembles any day of the week.

Work with it: So you've got a "prominent" rear. Maybe you have great legs or killer arms. As much as I would like you to have full body acceptance, there still may be some areas that you refuse to accept. If that is the case, show off the good stuff and move the focus away from the body parts you're too crazy to learn to love. Why waste energy on somehow improving this body part if there is nothing feasible you can do to change it? Life is too short for such silliness. If you hate anything from the hips down, wear something that flows away from the hips, like a fuller skirt or flat-front pants. If you hate your tummy, wear an empire waist top. If you hate your arms, wear a three-quarter-length sleeve.

Work it! Sometimes what we loathe about our bodies is not as bad as we think it is. Maybe, just maybe, if you focus on the part you hate and rock it like you love it, that feeling of hatred will go away. Remember Ricki's exposure therapy? When she was forced to face the very thing she feared, eventually the fear lessened and went away. Go ahead and call me crazy, but "working it" really works.

Balance the focus: Proportion is the key to dressing well. An oversized top with oversized pants will make you look like a blob. Stick to one oversized piece, if you must. This balancing rule also applies to clothing that is too tight, too long, too short, too plain, or too colorful. Mix it up to add interest and make your body look better.

Move to action: You can sit around feeling bad about yourself, or you can do something to change. Don't wait for your daughter to make the phone call! Nothing drives me more insane than people reading about change, asking about change, researching change, and hoping to change, but never acting to change. If your concerns about your body are healthy, not ones based in misperception or distortion, go ahead and get assistance, whether that means hiring a clothing consultant like me, getting to the gym, taking nutrition classes, or seeing your physician. If you don't like it, work to fix it. Sometimes just confronting what you don't like is as powerful and life-changing as the change itself. You'll see when you get there.

Take the time to outfit yourself beautifully and change your self-response. Rather than ignore your appearance, begin to act in a way that supports that you are worth more, even if you do not feel that way.

When you don't feel attractive, lovable, or accepted, remember to act as if you are beautiful, intelligent, worthy, and valuable. And how would a beautiful, intelligent, worthy, and valuable person behave? First and foremost, that person would take the time to choose a fabulous outfit to wear, style his or her hair, and choose wonderful accessories. Don't save your nice outfits for a party . . . wear them to the grocery store! Nothing is better than wrapping yourself in wonderful fabrics, catching your reflection, and being happy at what you see. Nurture your outer self to alter your response to your inner self . . . act as if!

Dressing for Your Body Type

No matter what your size and shape are, all bodies can be dressed to perfection. As much as I would love for you to be perfectly content in the shape you have and to dress in what you love rather than for the body part you hate, I know that may not be realistic. Still, there are ways to maximize and minimize what you deem to be "problem" areas.

The Top Part of Your Body

How to Minimize

A supportive bra is your first line of defense. You should find one that fully contains and supports you. If your breasts are toppling out of the cups, not only is that how they'll appear in a fitted shirt, but when you bend over your breasts will literally fall out of your bra. The back band of the bra should lie straight across without riding up or creating back overhang, the cups should lie flat against your body, and the straps should not dig into your shoulders. I would highly suggest getting a professional bra fitting!

Crossover styles, wraps, and V-necks accentuate your top half and often eliminate gaping and pulling fabrics. If you are uncomfortable with cleavage, buy layering tanks for modesty.

How to Maximize

You can choose to wear a bra or leave it at home. If you want some extra help, try a padded bra or gel inserts. Avoid clothing that is too loose around the bust, such as those with built-in seams or cups. Wear fitted boatnecks or crewnecks. If you want to appear bustier, try ruffles, extra material, or layered jewelry on top. You can also wear the deep-plunge styles seen frequently in formal attire.

The Middle of Your Body

How to Minimize

If you feel uncomfortable with your tummy or hips, there are many support garments that will smooth your middle, making dressing less traumatic. If you are choosing separates, try a loose top with fitted pants or a top that flares right under the bust. Dresses and tops that gather, ruche, or wrap at the middle can camouflage problem areas.

How to Maximize
Layering with separates adds bulk to the middle. If you want to accentuate curves, try adding a chunky belt or a skinny cinched belt to create the illusion of a smaller waist and larger hips. Flat-front high-waisted pants will accentuate your petite middle.

The Bottom of Your Body

How to Minimize
Make sure your undergarments fit smoothly, creating a seamless look once you put on your clothes. Wear pants that fit the largest part of your hips and rear and fall straight from that point. Make sure that your bottoms are not too loose, as they will conceal the curves of your body. If you feel uncomfortable in pants or fitted skirts, try a flared skirt with a flattering top.

How to Maximize
Avoid pants that sag or hang at the rear. You can wear very fitted styles, but if you would like to add more bulk, try a pleated skirt or wide-leg pants. There are garments with built-in padding in the seat to add curves where you need them.

Placing undue focus, judgment, and dissatisfaction on your body is an unnecessary exercise. The most essential part of you is intangible; your body is nothing more than its container.

A Note on Body Dysmorphic Disorder

Ricki struggled with poor body image, but fortunately her negative feelings did not reach levels that would have warranted clinical diagnosis and intervention. Body dysmorphic disorder (BDD), according to the *Diagnostic and Statistical Manual of Mental Disorders* (*DSM-IV-TR*), is a psychological disorder characterized by excessive concern about and preoccupation with perceived defects or minor deficits in one's physical features. This disorder occurs in 1 to 2 percent of the population.*

Those afflicted with this disorder may focus on one feature, many specific features, or their general appearance in ways that cause distress and impair social, occupational, and interpersonal functioning. In her study examining five hundred patients with BDD, Dr. Katharine Phillips, author of *The Broken Mirror,* found that the most commonly perceived deficits are with the nose, skin, and hair.** This disorder may often be part of an anxiety or eating disorder, or it may lead to depressive and anxiety disorders.

Those with BDD will think about their "flaws" at least once a day, often for hours at a time. They will obsessively check their appearance and/or cover their perceived flaws. These overwhelming fears about their appearance leave those who suffer with BDD fearful that others will notice their flaws. According to the *DSM-IV-TR,* BDD sufferers avoid possible criticism and ridicule by limiting or removing interactions with others from their lives, and they have difficulty functioning throughout the day.

---

* American Psychiatric Association (APA), *Diagnostic and Statistical Manual of Mental Disorders,* 4th ed., rev. (Washington, DC: APA, 2000).
** Katharine A. Phillips, MD, *The Broken Mirror: Understanding and Treating Body Dysmorphic Disorder* (New York: Oxford University Press, 2005).

As with most psychological disorders, BDD has multiple causes, including genetic and environmental factors that impact the individual's biological and psychological reactions. BDD symptoms usually occur equally in men and women and tend to arise in adolescence and early adulthood, a time when people generally are beginning to take note of and assess their external appearance.

BDD is treated with medication and/or psychotherapy. Because of its chronicity, untreated BDD will only persist or worsen. Women are more likely to seek treatment than men. Treatment is essential owing to the disorder's distressing symptoms as well as its high risk of suicidality.

If you have BDD or know someone who does, you can begin to find help at the websites for the American Psychological Association (http://www.apa.org), the American Psychiatric Association (http://www.psych.org), Mental Health America (http://www.nmha.org), or the National Institute of Mental Health (http://www.nimh.nih.gov).

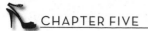

CHAPTER FIVE

Your Cover's Blown

When You Bare Too Much

I received a frantic message from Kate on a Thursday night. In a shaky voice, she requested an appointment during the weekend for an emergency makeover. She said that she was even willing to pay extra for my time on a weekend. When I called her back, Kate began, in a muffled whimper, to tell her story.

"During lunch today, my boss called me into her office to discuss my job performance. After going through her review, she told me that she wanted to discuss my attire. Some of our clients had made comments to her about what I wear! Including what I wore today. They felt it was too sexy for the office. Now my boss wants me to find some quote 'appropriate' clothes, or I can't go back to work on Monday. Can you believe this?"

Actually, I could. I see people all the time dressing inappropriately for any and all occasions, and they are often unaware that they are doing so.

When I arrived for the appointment, Kate came to the door in black high-heeled clogs, black leggings, and a black bra peeking out from under a white tank top. If this was what she wore to meet me for a makeover, I could just imagine what she wore to the office. "Hi, Kate," I said. Let's get right to it. Take me to your closet."

Her clothes were an adolescent girl's dream: bright pastels, glitter, minis, leggings, tank tops, belly shirts, and stilettos. Unfortunately, Kate was not an adolescent. She was a twenty-six-year-old woman.

We cleared out the closet and dumped all of the contents on the largest and cleanest surface we could find for navigating an effective purging. That turned out to be the floor of Kate's basement.

"Okay, Kate, I need to ask: what was the outfit you wore that got you into trouble?" I said. From the pile Kate picked out a ruche white button-down, a Hervé Ledger black band skirt, and sky-high red patent stilettos. "I love it," she said. "I don't know what's wrong with these people. What am I, a nun?"

I asked Kate to put the outfit on, so we could take a look.

Kate teetered toward me in the sky-high heels. I can certainly appreciate a beautiful shoe, but these needed a matching pole. Her body-hugging skirt left little to the imagination, including the lace thong underneath. The white button-down, the one item I had thought would be conservative enough for wearing to work, was unbuttoned low enough to reveal a seemingly endless line of cleavage. I could see why she had attracted attention.

Why We Show Skin: The Power of a Woman's Body

Before I became a psychologist, I was a teacher. One of my favorite exercises with preteen and teen female audiences was to ask them to look through magazine ads and tell me what was valued in women and what was valued in men. The magazines ranged from *Money* to *Teen Cosmo*. These little girls, with their fresh, pubescent minds, consistently came up with the same response. Women were valued for their youth (no wrinkles, glowing skin, and so on), beauty (big eyes, small nose, full lips, luxurious hair), and bodies (thin limbs, long legs, round bottom, large breasts, small waist). Men were valued for their success (expensive suit and watch, sports car, large home, job title, and so on).

A description of feminine characteristics often starts with our bodies. Ample breasts, curvy hips, small waist, and a plump backside are part of the female "ideal." As countless research studies have concluded, men are biologically driven to respond to the small waist-to-hip ratio of an hourglass figure. This magical ratio indicates that a female has the high levels of estrogen, fertility, and health that will make her the perfect partner for the male who wants to pass his genes to the next generation.

Throughout the millennia, female power has often been dependent on women's ability to bring offspring into the world, which depends in turn on the youthfulness of their bodies. As women age, their reproductive capacity disappears along with the markers of fertility: the magic hourglass ratio, the long, luscious locks, the soft, glowing skin.

So how do we grapple with age-old understandings of who we are in this modern world of women's liberation? Do we harness the power of the external, primarily our sexuality? Or do we focus on the internal, often at the cost of our sexuality? Are we able to have both?

When I was studying to become a psychologist, I learned about the social-psychological concept of the *Madonna-whore complex,* which describes the precarious decision that all women are forced to make. According to this theory, perceptions of women put them in two mutually exclusive categories: a female is either the sexless prude a man can take home to Mama or the super-slut he can "bed." Although we would like to think of our society as a forward-thinking one, these perceptions are present to this day—women are still perceived as either prude or slut by many men . . . and by many other women. The message sent by our clothing is usually the first information others receive about us, and it is this information they use to place us in these categories. If we are confronted on a daily basis with difficult wardrobe choices, being unable to identify a middle ground between those two options is often one of the reasons.

So how do you know how much is too much? In this chapter, you will learn how to identify the messages you are sending others with your clothes, the reasons for revealing, and the perfect balance between sexy and appropriate.

Could You Be Revealing Too Much?
A Checklist

- ☐ Do you wear the same size even though you have gained weight or grown taller?
- ☐ Are your clothes pulling at the seams?
- ☐ Are your clothes pulling at areas of closure, such as buttons, zippers, snaps, or hooks?
- ☐ Are your clothes bunching, buckling, or riding up?
- ☐ Are your clothes stretching over specific body parts?
- ☐ Are you unable to bend, lean, sit, or cross your legs without exposure?
- ☐ Are you wearing the same items to work as you are for nights out?
- ☐ Are you exposing cleavage?
- ☐ Are you exposing your belly button?
- ☐ Are you exposing your backside?
- ☐ Are you exposing your upper thighs?

- ❏ Are you exposing these body parts all at once?
- ❏ Do you find that men and women are staring at your exposed body?
- ❏ Do you find that your outfits attract negative or unwanted attention from men and women?
- ❏ Are you uncomfortable with this attention?
- ❏ Do you use body exposure as a means of attracting attention?
- ❏ Have you been told by family, friends, or coworkers that you need to "cover up" or "tone down" your outfits?
- ❏ Are you exposing more than others in the room?
- ❏ Have you ever been embarrassed that you exposed too much?
- ❏ Have you tried to change your look?
- ❏ When you cover up, do you feel unattractive?
- ❏ Are you having difficulty achieving the balance between sexy and demure?

If you have answered yes to many of these questions, you may be exposing too much. If you are comfortable with your level of exposure or it has not caused any negative consequences, this chapter is not for you. If you are uncomfortable but cannot find the balance between sexy and sweet, keep reading. This chapter will help you find the perfect look, examine the internal reasons for why you dress the way you do, and identify those inner qualities that are worth baring.

Case Study: How Kate Showed More When She Exposed Less

As we looked through Kate's clothes to bag the ripped, stained, and never-worn items, I had a chance to quickly assess her fashion choices. Although her clothes were often too short, too tight, or too revealing, Kate's overall aesthetic was quite sophisticated. For example, the infamous outfit she wore to the office, if tweaked, could have been incredibly classic. I made four observations about Kate's fashion choices, and as I identified the problem with them I also began to see the solution.

Observation 1:   Kate wore the same clothes to work, church, dinner, and clubbing.

    Problem: Kate did not differentiate clothing for various occasions. Whatever worked for the club, she seemed to believe, worked for everything else.

    Solution: Find basics that would work for all occasions. Discard or shelve clothes that worked only for situation-specific events and not others.

Observation 2:   The majority of Kate's clothes were saturated in Easter egg pastels.

    Problem: Pastels used with a light hand are attractive, but a wardrobe primarily in pastels can appear childish.

    Solution: Use pastels as accents, while using neutrals and more saturated colors as the wardrobe backbone.

Observation 3:   Kate's clothes did not fit her.

    Problem: They were often too short and too tight for her body.

    Solution: Learn what silhouettes properly fit her frame, including length, size, and coverage.

Observation 4:   Kate's clothes and accessories were highly embellished.

    Problem: Too much bling cheapened Kate's classy look.

    Solution: Find tasteful embellishments, to be used sparingly.

Unfortunately, Kate did not immediately recognize that her clothing choices were problematic. She believed that everyone else was "too damned uptight." My job was to find out why Kate took her innate Fifth Avenue sense of style to a Daytona spring break wet T-shirt contest.

Later that afternoon, I asked Kate to wear her favorite outfit on a trip downtown. On top, she wore a deep V-neck hot pink shirt with a zebra-print padded bra exposed. On the bottom, stretch pants in nice translucent white, no underwear required. Kate's job was just to walk through the stores to browse and shop.

While Kate was busy browsing, I solicited the opinions of other shoppers regarding her ensemble. I recorded each response on a note card that I would read to Kate at a later time. After the shopping trip, Kate and I returned to the house to discuss the excursion.

I asked Kate what she thought about her outfit and what message she thought it might be sending to others. Her first response was "Message? What message?" Kate did not realize that her clothing said anything at all. I went through the opinion cards with her: "Not appropriate." . . . "Is she going to a club?" . . . "Slutty." . . . "Does her mother know about this?" . . . "Oh yeah, that's hot." . . . "Trashy!" . . . "I'd take that."

I didn't mince words when I relayed this commentary. In the period of silence that followed, Kate's face flushed, and she began to cry. "I'm not a slut! What am I supposed to wear? Just because I am twenty-six, does that mean I have to look ugly? I don't want to look ugly!"

Billboard Theory:
Understanding How Others View Us

People read our outside to see who we are on the inside, and what others read in Kate's clothing was "inappropriate" and "sleazy." Since that wasn't how Kate felt about herself, there was an incongruence between her outer and inner selves. My job was to make the inside and outside match. Kate needed to embrace her entire self with appropriate clothing, and to also project a message to the outside world that she had chosen herself.

Like it or not, we are often categorized, or we categorize others, in certain ways depending on our clothing choices. If a woman wears a classic sheath with a strand of pearls, she is categorized as successful. If she wears a raggedy sweatshirt, she is seen as not in control of her life. If she wears a revealing outfit, we think, she must crave attention.

Although we may fight against this tendency to categorize, it's human nature that drives us to put people, places, and things in neatly labeled boxes. If you dress like a prep (embroidered pants, rep ties, lax flow, and so on), others will assume not only that you belong to the prep group but that you have all the qualities of a prep: you spend your summers on your yacht, you are legacy Ivy League, your home is filled with antiques, and your last name is followed by a Roman numeral.

We make these assumptions because they take the least amount of effort. Our preference for *generalization* follows from our preference for *parsimony*. Parsimony is the use of the simplest answer to explain something. Looking at a person, examining his style, and placing him in the most obvious category takes little to no effort and seems to us to make the most sense.

Kate was confronted with the pain of parsimony. After our trip downtown, Kate found that she had immediately been categorized by people who saw her. These observers had assessed Kate's outfit as that of an "easy" girl; therefore, using the simplest explanation, that was what Kate must be.

Uncovering the Past

I asked Kate *when* she started wearing her signature sexy look. "When I had the body to wear them," Kate responded. "Probably during puberty, like twelve."

I then asked Kate *why* she started wearing the look. Kate stated that she had "overdeveloped" quickly. "I was twelve with the body of a woman." Here, I saw, was the root of the internal trauma influencing her clothing choices.

Boys who develop early find that they are at a social, sexual, emotional, and psychological advantage. Whereas boys' development and outcome are directly proportional, for girls the relationship is indirect. When a girl develops too much too soon, she is at a strong disadvantage. Early development often decreases her academic performance, social adjustment, and self-esteem.[*] As a woman, Kate wasn't the hot football player that all the guys admired and the girls loved: she was the "girl with the big boobs" who got her bra strap snapped. This early experience left Kate with a love-hate relationship with her body. She loved the power it had over others and the attention it received, yet hated that her intelligence and humor were ignored, and she didn't always know how to manage the effects of her figure on those around her.

Kate was a little girl trapped in a big girl's body, like a child driving a car. She hadn't learned how to drive, stop, go, follow the signs, know where she was going, and avoid bad drivers. Kate had been given a super-sized dose of feminine power and had no idea how to harness it.

---

[*] B. M. Newman and P. R. Newman, *Development Through Life: A Psychosocial Approach* (Belmont, CA: Wadsworth Cengage Learning, 2006).

Like many girls going through early puberty, Kate had the difficult task of acquiring a woman's body with the mind of a child. "I was so uncomfortable going through puberty. I remember looking at myself in the mirror and thinking *What is happening to me?* Some girls halt puberty by refusing to eat, or they start to cover their new bodies. Others, like Kate, choose to overcompensate for their discomfort through overexposure. Both options are ineffective attempts to gain control.

Accustomed to lots of attention, Kate said she learned that she did not receive attention when she covered herself. Ultimately, she decided that exposing would be her means of coping with the changes in her body she could not stop. Although this sounded like the answer to Kate's issue of overexposure, I believed that Kate's behaviors were rooted in something much deeper.

Overt, excessive, underdeveloped, or unhealthy sexual expression can be the result of a *sexual, psychological insult*. This ranges from receiving a criticism about a body part as a child to being sexually harassed by a family member. The sexual expression born out of trauma may initially serve a functional purpose, whether protecting the body from viewing (covering) or fulfilling unmet internal needs with external acts (overexposure). When the trauma has passed and the person is left with only a traumatic memory, the coping mechanisms that once saved her in the past, no longer work in the present. They have not only lost their purpose but arrested her development. She is coping with something that no longer exists and engaging in behaviors that keep her stuck in the past.

Every look, sneer, and catcall reminded Kate of the incongruence between her emotional maturity and her physical maturity. "Your body was made just for sex" was one of the many crude comments that haunted Kate. She coped with this objectification the best way she knew how—by, ironically, exaggerating her sexuality. Showing more of her body enabled her to control some aspect of the situation.

Unfortunately, as she grew older Kate never changed her strategy and continued dressing like an adolescent who looked like a woman but wasn't one.

The Downtown Experiment

It was a Friday night, and Kate and I were going to go where the men were: happy hour. I asked Kate to wear her hottest outfit. She put on her tight jeans, light pink shoes, light pink lace lingerie top, and her favorite item, the water bra. She threw on her diamond hoops, bangles, a rhinestone watch, and a ring for almost every finger.

This was a perfect opportunity for me to observe Kate in her natural habitat. "Kate, I want to see you in action. I want to see just what kind of attention you get tonight." Predictably, as the night went on, that attention amounted to pats on her rear end, comments about her cleavage, and plenty of dirty stares from women. Kate gave out her number repeatedly, had plenty of free drinks, and even received multiple invitations to spend the night.

On Saturday morning, Kate and I discussed the night. "So, Kate, is that usually the kind of attention you get?" "Yeah," Kate replied. "The guys love me!"

"Kate, you said you were looking for a relationship." I couldn't resist asking. "How many of the guys who ask for your number call you? Has any one of them turned into a long-term relationship or deeper connection?"

"Not really," Kate replied, indifferently. "But I'm young and have time to find a good one."

After a long pause, Kate said, "Well, I guess I would like a nice guy, but I don't think they exist."

A few weeks later, Kate and I got ready for our second night out, but this time I dressed her. I pulled out the Hervé Leger black band skirt and paired it with a sleeveless crewneck black silk tank. I had Kate tuck the shell into the skirt to create a bloused effect. The waist was finished with a black patent belt to match her black patent shoes. She was allowed one piece of jewelry, which was a pair of large diamond studs.

We headed out to the same lounge where we had spent that first Friday night. This time Kate turned quite a few heads, but no one leered, stared, or ogled. She had her chair pulled out for her and her door opened, but did not get prodded, poked, or grabbed. By the end of the night, no one had asked for her number, bought her a drink, or invited her home, but she did have a wonderful conversation with one man and was invited to dance with a group of women celebrating an impending wedding.

Kate enjoyed her night out and even was relieved that she could "just have fun without worrying about getting guys." Having men want to speak to her and capturing their interest with her conversation as much as her outfit felt good.

Using the external self, such as your sparkling eyes, fantastic legs, or shiny hair, to enhance the internal self can be a successful technique for improving social experience. Using external qualities as the sole technique for social interaction, however, only teaches us to focus on the outside. Kate felt that all she had to give others was "a little thigh here and a lot of cleavage there." She completely discounted all of her unique internal qualities, which were far more attractive and meaningful.

Physical attraction is usually the initial force that brings couples together, but it isn't the glue that holds them together. I pointed out the obvious to Kate: since our looks change as we get older, what did she think was going to happen when she couldn't rely on the "hot bod of a twenty-six-year-old" anymore?

After this experiment, Kate and I discussed what she had learned. "I always thought that my dressing choices were limited to extremes;

that they had to be dramatic. You know, prude or slut, boring or hot. Now I know that there is a middle ground."

I wanted Kate to dig a little deeper. "What else did you learn from this?" I asked her.

"I guess I want to be noticed for more than my breasts. I mean, I definitely didn't get as much attention as I normally do the night you dressed me, but it was quality over quantity." I explained to Kate that her clothing might appear to draw attention but actually distracted from the view. "Kate, no one really sees you in the clothing," I told her. "They just see the parts and pieces."

Though she initially resisted, Kate finally understood that covering more did not take away from her value or the likelihood that someone would find her attractive. She decided that the attention she received when exposed was not going to help her form the deeper emotional connection with someone that she was looking for. "Okay, Dr. B, I get it now. But the toughest part is finding the balance between looking trashy and looking uptight."

I smiled. "Kate, this is the easy part. We just need to have the internal you match the you that you show to the world." Kate's appearance did not convey the appropriate message she wanted to send. Our next task was to formulate Kate's message and have her dress the part.

Tailoring the Message

"I just want to feel young and hot in my outfits," Kate said. "I want to show off my curves. . . . I mean, if I am going to spend an hour on the treadmill every day, I want to show off my hard work."

I had to take a step back. "I hear you, Kate, but what do you want to say about yourself?"

Kate thought for a minute, then said, "I want to look young, sleek, fun, and professional. I want to look like I can run the company and still melt a man's heart." I knew what Kate wanted, and it was a familiar trope—Kate wanted to be a "power woman."

"Yes!" Kate exclaimed. "That's what I want, Dr. B. I want to say: 'I am a *power* woman.'"

Realizing her potential power, or desire for it, was especially important to Kate's progress. Like some women (though not all), Kate actually lost the very power she sought by overexposing. Using her body as an object and putting it all out there did not come from a place of power but rather from a place of vulnerability. When she wore barely there styles, her look was a plea for approval: "Look at this! Do you find this attractive?" The desperation of her hope that everyone looking at her would say, "Yeah!" was painfully apparent. By contrast, when you dress like a "power woman," you dress in a manner that shows appreciation for your body. Whether or not you get a response is inconsequential.

Kate was lucky that she had many great classic pieces in her wardrobe that, worn properly, would give her the look and convey the message she desired. We created many outfits from the basics in her closet: fitted dark jeans with a simple white tank for casual wear; a sleek black skirt suit with a hint of lace underneath; and a cream fitted sheath with an animal print belt.

In time Kate was finally able to identify the message she had been sending and then re-create her wardrobe to send a different message, one suited to her ideal representation as a "power woman" and in line with her own self-declared attributes of being "generous" and "artistic." Kate still maintained her sexy self, but remained professional and tasteful. And more and more, she enjoyed the company of men rather than the objectification she had received from some of them.

Most importantly, she solved the initial crisis she'd had at work: her boss congratulated her on the improvements to her attire. Kate even reported that she felt more qualified for her job because she dressed like she was. She admitted that it did take her some time to "turn down the volume" and get used to the "decreased stares." But after just a few weeks, Kate discovered that the quality of attention she received was far more important than the quantity.

Your Turn

Get the Message

Through the "downtown" experiment, Kate examined the message her clothing sent to others and thought about whether this message matched the one she wanted to project. If you are looking for a supplement to this exercise, or a less extreme option, look no further than a large stack of fashion magazines.

As a psychologist, I frequently use magazines with patients to examine messages about gender roles, equality, identity formation, and sexuality. Analyzing the messages conveyed by the clothing in magazines develops a skill that we can then use to analyze our own wardrobes. Most of us are better able to analyze others than ourselves, which explains why therapists never lack for patients. A therapist helps patients develop the objective eye that they eventually internalize. I hoped that Kate would use other-analysis, through magazines, to facilitate her own analysis and eventually internalize my message.

To do this experiment, begin by examining the outfits in your magazines. Try to identify the messages that each outfit is sending. If you find it difficult to do this, invite a friend or family member over to participate. The more people the better in fact, since then you'll have a consensus.

Like Kate, you will be able to expertly identify each message that clothing items send about the wearer—including your own items—by the end of this exercise. Move to your clothing pile and lay out the outfits you're thinking about wearing. Analyze the message they are sending. Like Kate, you will see that small tweaks in your outfits can create large changes in the overall message.

Now it's time to clean the slate and create outfits for the new you!

Create the Message

What woman doesn't love to be admired, to feel attractive, to know that she's "got it"? In an effort to have this experience, we may go shorter, tighter, and hotter. Sadly, there is no empowerment in this approach. Just because we are old enough to choose to use our sexuality in whatever way we see fit does not mean that our choice is always coming from a place of liberation and power. If we believe that our only value is in our ability to use our sexuality to entice men, then it is only through external feedback that we find internal worth. And that puts us right back in the days when our bodies were stuffed into corsets.

Finding a balance is necessary when toning down exposure or showing a little more. Creating a look that incorporates elements of sexy can be a difficult task, but there are steps to navigate the process.

Function: From the original analysis, I taught Kate to identify the basics in her wardrobe that worked for all occasions and those clothes that only worked for situation-specific events. Kate's white button-down, black pencil skirt, tanks, blazers, patent heels, and belts were multi-functional. Her strappy sandals, miniskirts, and fitted tops were appropriate only for nights out. We placed these latter items together in a separate space in her closet.

Your most functional clothes are easy to identify. They are the ones you wear all the time, wash on a weekly basis, or feel at a loss for a replacement if left too long in the hamper. Your classics should work for you during most seasons and for most functions, and they should mix well with other pieces. These "can't live without" items should fit you properly (not too tight or short), be made in a color that makes your skin glow, and be crafted in a fabric that withstands the test of time and a rigorous wash.

Color: I removed many of Kate's basic clothing pieces—shoes, pants, dresses—that were pastel and bordering on teenage cutesy. I kept the smaller pastel items, such as her scarves, summer tops, and jewelry, and we went shopping for jewel-toned clothing to replace the basic pieces. Kate recognized that her wardrobe was stuck in adolescence because she had still not worked through her adolescent trauma issues. Once I showed Kate that her wardrobe was enabling her to remain stuck, she was willing to make some changes. And she was eventually willing to confront the deeper stuff with a therapist.

Like Kate, you too can choose colors that convey the message you have decided to send. All colors have a specific mood-inducing effect.

Red is the color of power, danger, and aggression . . . think stop signs, red lights, blood, and the red carpet. This strong color increases appetite, heart rate, breathing, and the attention of others. Red clothing often connotes strength, femininity, and sexuality.

Orange makes us feel warmth, health, and change. It is often associated with the fall holidays, Halloween and Thanksgiving, and the harvest time. Because orange is the contrasting color of blue, it is used for safety clothing and equipment to stand out against the surrounding sky.

Yellow jolts the senses and in large quantities can overwhelm. In addition to increasing concentration, yellow can push us overboard and increase agitation. In fashion, yellow is often used in small doses, as it can be harsh on the skin.

Green, the color of nature, relaxes, makes us feel refreshed, and is associated with things that produce. Think money, fertility, and green traffic lights!

Blue is one of the most common colors on our planet. From the ocean to the sky, the color blue cradles us in its calming hue. It can also indicate sadness: we have all heard the expression "feeling blue."

Purple, the color of pomp, circumstance, and royalty, oozes sophistication and glamour. This color is often used during the fall and winter months. To modernize the color, use it with other brights.

White equals purity and sterility. This color is clean, clear, and goes with everything. It has traditionally been an indicator of high status because keeping it clean required a life of leisure and the help to maintain its purity. White reflects all the colors of the chromatic spectrum, which is especially important during the summer months.

Black has often been associated with dark forces. It has a connotation of power as well as submission. Despite its negative associations, black is the most popular color in fashion for its classic appeal, slimming effect, and ability to work well with all other colors. Little black dress, anyone?

Fit and Proportion: You can have the most exquisite clothes in the world, but if they don't fit, the outfit is ruined. I took Kate to a tailor to teach her appropriate fit for various garments, particularly length. If you find that your movement is hindered by fear of exposure, your clothes are too short. When your clothes are the appropriate length, bending, leaning over, and sitting should not reveal your underwear. Whether you are trying on old clothes in your closet or new ones in the store, make sure you can sit, stand, bend, lean, and squat without hesitation.

If your clothes are too tight, you will often see rippling at the bust, back, thighs, and rear. Clothing should not buckle, bunch, or ride up when you move. If it does, it's too tight! Closures such as buttons, zippers, snaps, and hooks should lie flat; if they are pulling or gaping, your clothes are too tight. Always buy clothes that fit the largest part of you and have the other areas altered. If you have a large chest, find a top that fits it. If your arms are too large, have the garment tailored to fit that area. Remember: you can always make a garment smaller, but not larger. Most seams have only a one- to two-inch allowance, which is not enough for significant alterations.

When you wear fitted pieces, keep the look smooth. The days of wearing biker shorts under our clothes are over. You can find support garments for any cut, length, fabric, or size. Whether you are wearing plunge or halter, skintight or oversized, bulky or sheer, there is something available. Just as I did with Kate, you should look through your clothes and make a list of the foundation pieces you will need to wear with each item. For example, a strapless dress requires a strapless bra. A satin gown requires a smoother. Bring your clothes with you when shopping for foundation garments to make sure that everything fits properly.

After each piece has been carefully tailored and matched with appropriate undergarments, you can mix and match tops and bottoms to create all of your looks. When dressing, use the fashion balance principle I swear by, for every figure: loose on the top, tight on the bottom; tight on the top, loose on the bottom; revealing on the top, covered on the bottom; revealing on the bottom, covered on the top; and so forth. This ensures perfect proportions and balanced ensembles.

Accessories: After your closet is stocked with underwear appropriate for your clothes, don't forget to accessorize. If you keep your clothing classic, simple, and unadorned, all you need to do to change your look is change your accessories. This strategy saves time, money, and closet space while guaranteeing that you are always in style.

Changing your accessories is also an easy way to experiment with demure or sexy styles. For example, a modest turtleneck sweater dress can become alluring with fishnet stockings or over-the-knee-leather boots. A deep V-neck dress can be worn over a button-down and pearls, or a lace cami with diamond hoops.

Remember to embellish effectively and efficiently. Using one accessory as a focus of interest creates a greater impact than cluttering the body with a bunch of junk. As Madame Chanel said, "When accessorizing, always take off the last thing you put on."

Investing in one exquisite piece in your accessories collection is far better than wasting money on many subpar pieces. I took Kate on a trip to the store to teach her how to identify the natural materials, proper construction, and classic designs that go into quality accessories. If you are having trouble finding accessories to invest in, find inspiration in magazines and get information from sales professionals.

Quick Tips for
Covering Up to Show Yourself

Start out easy: The way to build lasting self-esteem is to accomplish tasks that guarantee success. To use your gifts and talents in a way that helps others is the best way to maximize your internal rewards. When you pay attention to the external qualities, while helping others, your success is guaranteed.

Then make it a little harder: Set low-level challenges that you are likely to meet, such as taking a class or running a half-marathon. Increase the difficulty level as you accomplish each goal. The more successes you have, the more willing you will be to try more difficult challenges.

Look to others: Start focusing on the positives in others. It takes a greater level of self-esteem to pay less attention to yourself and more to others and their accomplishments.

Accentuate the attribute you love most about yourself: If it's your eyes, try a smoky eye or fake eyelashes. Maybe you like your legs—so go for the shorter skirt or shorts.

Achieve balance in your exposure: If you are showing a lot of leg, don't let it all hang out up top. If your top is bursting, wear pants or a longer skirt.

Consider your audience and your comfort level with them: The skimpy shorts may not feel so comfortable when you are dancing at a fraternity house. The inflate-a-bra may not be the right choice for your boyfriend's family celebration.

Consider the message you are sending with your outfit: Are you really shocked that everyone is staring at your cleavage all night when your breasts are screaming *Look at me!* in a shirt made of mesh? Are you really surprised that no one has even asked you out when you always wear bulky sweater dresses? Rather than complain about people's reactions after the fact, claim accountability for the look you go out with.

Consider the outcome you want: If you want to be objectified, by all means put on the *Baywatch*-inspired outfit. If you want to be appreciated, wear the Marilyn Monroe white dress and diamond cuff. And if you want to be ignored, throw on a mother superior robe.

Don't Forget the Power of the Stiletto

We have become experts at using our clothing and fashion accessories to enhance all that we are as females and to attract attention. While some pieces get attention for all of the wrong reasons, such as the much-loved booty short, others enhance our femininity without giving it all away. Nothing says female more than the high heel. If you want to instantly feel sexier without the compromise, slip on a stiletto.

The negative connotation of the high heel has certainly changed. These shoes were once regarded as an implement of torture or control. We need only look back at the ancient Chinese ritual of binding the feet. Purportedly intended to increase femininity, bound feet ultimately removed a woman's ability to move freely. There are those who still argue that the heel only serves to constrain the female, but I find that I can walk, run, and jump far better in a heel than a flat. There are those who argue that the heel leaves a woman defenseless. Try and catch me and you may find a four-inch stiletto jammed in your eye!

Heels are now a symbol of female power and sensuality. By emphasizing the strength of the calf, the tilt of the hip, and the thrusting outward of the derriere, heels accentuate female sexuality. It has been hypothesized that the posture a woman takes when she's wearing heels mimics the posture of both human females and other female animals ready for sex, also known as *lordosis behavior*.

As sexually powerful as a high heel may make you feel, it serves another purpose as well: it creates physical power. When giving a presentation, meeting with a client, or making a pitch to a potential referral, that extra height boosts your confidence. With an average female height of five-foot-four, most of us are either shorter or the same height as most people in the room; with four-inch heels on, we are taller than everyone else. No one is looking at the tops of our heads—we are looking at theirs.

The sound and sight of high heels also create a lasting memory. The clicking of Manolos announces our arrival before we even enter the room, much like the medieval heralds with horns and banners preparing the way for the queen. And the visual memory of the heel is an effective way to make connections. "Oh, hello, future client. We met last week. My name is Ms. So-and-So, the one wearing the leopard print stilettos. Oh yes, of course you remember me!"

The Right Height

Even with all of its advantages, the heel has fallen prey to stereotypes against women. For example, some view heel height as proportional to a woman's promiscuity. They don't call them stripper shoes for nothing. So how can you pick the best heel height for yourself?

We turn to sports psychologist Yuri Hanin for the answer. He has proposed that athletes perform best at a specific level of anxiety that he calls the *zone of optimal state anxiety*. Since this level is different for every individual, each of us has an *individualized zone of optimal functioning*.* Now let's apply this idea to heel height.

Each woman has a heel height that allows her to perform at maximum capacity. This height is determined by her gross motor skills, her height, and, most importantly, her ability to confidently rock her heels. If you are teetering, tripping, covered in blisters, and barely

---

*Y. L. Hanin, "Emotions and Athletic Performance: Individual Zones of Optimal Functioning," *European Yearbook of Sport Psychology* 1(1997): 29–72.

able to walk, you have not achieved your optimal heel height. If you are shuffling around in flats like Howard Hughes with tissue boxes, you have not achieved your optimal heel height. Some women are born able to walk in skyscraper heels professionally, others must find a height somewhere in the middle, and others should stick to the training wheel of shoes, the flat.

The appropriate heel height may also depend on where you wear them. Look around you: are others wearing super-high shoes, or are you the only one? If you are the only one, is it because wearing heels at your hyperconservative job is inappropriate, or because you're short? Have your heels hindered either your physical movement (walking or standing all day) or your figurative movement (landing the next account or being taken seriously)?

Also analyze feedback from others when making an appropriate heel height choice. Do people stare at you? Do they compliment your choices? If your friends at work comment on your shoe choices without giving you an actual compliment, rethink your shoe. For example, "Oh, I knew that was you down the hall. All that clacking echoes in my head from a mile away." "Boy, it sure looks hard for you to walk in your shoes."

When shopping for your heels, strive to *achieve balance*. Consider pairing a higher heel with a more conservative fabric and style of heel and a longer-length skirt. If you have a higher heel with a crazy pattern, pair it with a more conservative outfit. Use a lower heel with a more provocative outfit, or power up a lower heel with a crazy pattern or silhouette. Always use *pumps to punctuate*. Remember, shoes are accessories. Make sure they enhance the outfit rather than detract from it. When used properly, the high heel can become the "sole" of your femininity.

Whether we wear sky-high stilettos or halter tops, our desire to feel attractive, accentuate our figures, and enjoy attention from others is healthy. However, when this desire leads us to dress inappropriately, sends faulty messages about who we are, and makes us dependent on the responses of others to determine our value, the consequences are not so healthy. A miniskirt and bikini top will never reveal our inner beauty, and nothing is sexier than that!

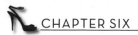

CHAPTER SIX

Adventures in Time Travel

When You Are
Not Dressing for Your Age

The Fear of Aging

Whether named outright or veiled in euphemism, fear of aging is a driving force in consumer habits. From plastic surgery to wrinkle creams, from preadolescents on catwalks to children on the pages of fashion magazines, the desire to halt aging or ease painful thoughts of it is ever present.

Perhaps we fear aging because we have a deep-seated fear of our mortality, which ultimately drives our survival instinct. If we always looked young, we would never see the effects of time, the reminders that our bodies are slowly breaking down. Aging may also include loss of functioning, pain, and isolation on the path to death. Depressing, I know! But when twenty-year-olds are getting Botox in their "wrinkles" and fifty-year-olds are getting butt implants because they "don't have the body they used to," are such panicked reactions against aging really necessary? Or even healthy?

A *phobia* is an intense, irrational fear of a stimulus coupled with irrational avoidance—the key word here being *irrational*. Our almost obsessive avoidance of our wrinkles, graying hair, age spots, hair loss, and varicose veins is reaching phobic levels. When I search for beauty, fashion, or health articles or shows online, on TV or in print, I am guaranteed to find extensive coverage of two topics: weight loss and aging. We are told that looking older is unattractive, we believe that, and then we buy things to defend ourselves against it.

As women, we are quite aware of what our bodies may experience, but this body focus is less on functioning and more on aesthetics as we take in messages about the depth of our wrinkles, the expansiveness of our cellulite, and the levels to which our skin may fall. Information about how to defy the aesthetic impact of aging is very easy to find, and we are quite expert at slowing the process.

Women often equate aging with a loss of beauty. From an evolutionary perspective, women are sexually attractive in their childbearing years. If a man believes he will be able to pass on his genetic material through a suitable female partner—one who can carry the child and provide the best genetic material—he will find her more attractive and mate with her. When females are no longer able to bear children, men no longer find us sexually desirable and will always prefer younger women.

Fortunately, female attraction goes beyond our baby-making capacity, but its association with youth, fertility, and beauty still haunts us as we get older. We may lie about our age or refuse to tell people. Those who proudly tout their age, such as celebrities, models, and socialites, often do so only after denying their nips, tucks, and injectibles. When they proceed to reprimand the rest of us for not being content with our own natural aging and suggest a few yoga poses, multivitamins, and sunscreen, it is hard not to feel insulted. Easy for them to say when they look like they just escaped from Madame Tussauds Wax Museum.

Many women believe that they lose their relevance or currency in this world when they feel that they have lost their looks. Just take note of what happens on the silver screen. Those once super-sexy goddesses of television and film are replaced by younger models. Older men can continue to play leading roles and maintain their sex symbol status with a much younger female co-star. In an attempt to win back her allure and some screen time, the older actress turns to plastic surgery, weight loss, and a style makeover. Though criticized for these attempts, she knows that if she did nothing she would be equally scrutinized for aging before our eyes!

Aging gracefully is a complicated process requiring change at both the internal and external levels. If you have been stuck dressing the same way through the years, have given up by dressing older than you are, or have given in by buying into the youth obsession, then this chapter is for you. You will learn to identify inappropriate age-dressing, examine the internal reasons for your behaviors, and find ways to improve your look.

Dressing Your Age

Many factors are involved in crafting the perfect ensemble—size, length, color, level of embellishment, appropriateness, function—and figuring out what to wear can be an overwhelming and difficult process. As we get older, our age becomes yet another factor to consider when deciding what to wear, what to give away, what to keep, and what to buy.

Acknowledging our age or the process of aging can be painful, but when we try to remain unaware of it, our look suffers. Those who have ignored their age in the dressing process make one of three mistakes: (1) they never change their look and dress the same way over the years, which makes them look out of touch and out of style; (2) they dress older than they are, figuring that, since we all have to age, they might as well do it their own way; or (3) they dress too young, which paradoxically ages them.

The only way to keep the same look for years is to trap ourselves in a time warp. If our look no longer works in the present, others will assume that everything else about us has become irrelevant as well. When we fatalistically dress older than we are in an attempt to control the inevitable, we are actually avoiding a true examination of the aging process by not acknowledging where we currently are in the process; instead, we are rushing through it and giving up prematurely on aging well. Finally, when we dress younger than we are in an attempt to hide our real age, we are actually drawing attention to it. When the look does not match the person, the incongruence is what other people see first.

Staying Current: A Checklist

Dressing the Same
- ❑ Do your yearbooks and old pictures reveal that your hairstyle was the same then as it is now? Your clothing choices? Your makeup?
- ❑ Have you kept your clothes for five years or more? Ten years or more?
- ❑ What percentage of your closet is composed of new items?
- ❑ What percentage of your closet is composed of old items (five to ten years old)?
- ❑ Do you find that you have worn a trend that has cycled through the fashion world more than once?

❏ Are your clothes composed of trends from another era, such as those from the '60s, '70s, '80s, or '90s?

❏ Have your friends or family suggested that you try a new look?

❏ Are you uncomfortable trying a new look?

❏ Are you unable to change your look?

❏ Do you resist incorporating current trends into your wardrobe?

❏ Are you afraid that if you change your look you will make a fashion error?

If you have answered yes to most of these questions, you may be stuck in a time warp. It is time to find out why you are stuck, lose your dated look, and move on internally.

Dressing Too Old

❏ Do you find that you do not dress like your peers?

❏ Are you wearing clothes similar to those of women in your mother's or grandmother's generation?

❏ Are you buying clothes in departments that cater to older women?

❏ Do people often think you are older than you are?

❏ Do you feel that you would not look good in styles meant for your age?

❏ Have you given up trying to age gracefully?

❏ Do you feel that, since aging is inevitable, why try to put any effort into your look?

❏ Is finding clothes for your age confusing to you?

❏ Has a friend or family member suggested that you change your look?

❏ Have you often rejected the fashion suggestions of others?

❏ Have you tried to change your look but are afraid to do so?

❏ Would you like to look different but don't know how to make the change?

If you have answered yes to most of these questions, you may be aging yourself. Find out why you are speeding up the process so that you can turn back the time on your closet.

Dressing Too Young

❑ Do you dress differently than your peers?

❑ Do you wear clothes from younger generations?

❑ Do you shop in the juniors section of the store or copy the styles from those departments?

❑ Do you follow the trends?

❑ Are you afraid that you will look like an "old lady"?

❑ Do you avoid telling people your age?

❑ Do you lie about your age?

❑ Do you find birthdays depressing?

❑ Do you use anti-aging products?

❑ Do you go to extreme measures to fight your age?

❑ Do you spend a large proportion of your income to fight the aging process?

If you answered yes to most of these questions, you may be dressing too young for your age. Learn how to accept where you are in the present and find a stylish, age-appropriate wardrobe to match.

Stuck in a Time Warp

All that was needed to accompany Brad's worn bell-bottom jeans, skintight polyester printed shirt, and medallion nestled in his chest hair was a disco ball. From his wardrobe to his Pinto, not much had changed for Brad since his thirties, which was almost forty years ago.

He still held his first job, remained single and rarely dated, and continued to live in his mother's large house after her death.

He came to me requesting assistance during the transitional period leading up to his retirement. After working with Brad for multiple sessions without making any progress toward significant change, including his attire, I addressed the meaning of change for Brad. Often when people resist an intervention in therapy, taking the indirect route leads to direct outcomes. For example, rather than working on a specific plan for dating or downsizing, Brad and I discussed the process of change, the important areas of change in his life, and his understanding of change as a positive or negative experience. It was in this analysis of change that I discovered the root of Brad's resistance to it and the solution to overcome it.

Brad experienced his first major and most traumatic change during childhood when his father died suddenly. Brad picked up the slack by taking care of anything that his mother was unable to handle. He did not have the luxury of making a career change, pursuing a relationship, or purchasing a home. All of the normal developmental peaks and troughs were never present in Brad's life. After his father's death, Brad's life was placed on cruise control. No turns, no detours, no speed bumps or obstacles—Brad just kept moving forward, never noticing the changing scenery around him.

Brad was willing to change but found it difficult to put this desire into an operational plan. One of the most immediate changes he could make was to update his wardrobe. Brad's biggest concern in this area was that he might come across as a "a dirty old man trying to look cool." One of the main reasons he did not change his '70s style was simply that he didn't know how to.

There is no better way to address a fear of change in a wardrobe than to introduce the classic pieces that will never change. A dress shirt, cufflinks, a cashmere sweater, a trench coat, fitted trousers, a cotton T-shirt, and a perfect pair of jeans provided a safe alternative to Brad's *Saturday Night Fever* look. We extended this safe and time-less approach to fashion in other areas of Brad's life. We approached the unfamiliar—such as dating, meeting new friends, leaving his job, finding a new apartment, and even buzzing off the comb-over—in ways that were familiar, conservative, and comfortable to Brad.

Even though Brad eliminated the majority of his dated wardrobe, he did keep his printed velour jumpsuit to wear once a year . . . for Halloween!

Helping Your Inner Brad

In psychology, stressors in life can be measured using what is called the Social Readjustment Rating Scale.* On this scale, life events are given a numerical value based on the level of stress they induce, from coping with the death of a spouse to enjoying a vacation. All of the items listed represent changes in the status quo, and any kind of change, positive or negative, inevitably creates stress in our lives. A healthy response requires adjustment, learning, assessment, and flexibility.

Often change, especially in the wardrobe, can leave us not only stressed but confused. Scratching our heads, we may ask: How do I know it's time for a change? When do I know my look has become outdated? How do I change to stay in style but not be trendy? How do I stay ahead of fashion but maintain a style appropriate for my age and lifestyle? You can take the following three steps to answer all of these questions.

---

* T. H. Holmes and R. H. Rahe, "The Social Readjustment Rating Scale," *Journal of Psychosomatic Research* 11(2, 1967): 213–218.

Identify: If you are anything like Brad, you may never know that you need a change until someone tells you that you do or it is forced upon you. One of the most obvious indicators of style stagnation is a wardrobe whose contents have remained exactly the same for more than five years. Although the catwalks change rapidly, fashion themes such as color, fit, length, and level of embellishment seem to hold for a few years . . . but they *do* expire eventually.

Inventory: Each season you should take inventory of your clothing to decide what can stay and what should go. Classics, such as those that Brad invested in, can always stay. Although you want to maintain the basic structure of your wardrobe, you can make subtle changes to classic pieces over the years. So update your classics with any sort of change that feels comfortable to you. For example, the white button-down will always be in style, but the length, the placement of the buttons, the size of the collar, and the fit will all change. This year you may want a fitted white button-down that is longer and has French cuffs, and next year you may want a boyfriend fit with three-quarter-length sleeves.

Reconsider: If you are still struggling with the idea of change, examine the components of your outdated clothing that you like. Maybe you like the bright red color of your '80s miniskirt, or the embroidered detail of your '50s poodle skirt. Then look for those components in updated pieces. Buy a bright red patent leather shoe or an embroidered T-shirt. Also note your patterns of dress. If you are a jacket-and-skirt kind of gal but your outfit is stuck in the early '90s, continue wearing skirts and jackets, but in updated silhouettes, fabrics, and colors. When it comes to your wardrobe, you can stay safe, but do it with style!

Dressing Too Old

From her clothing choices, no one would have guessed that Ginny was in her midthirties. The polyester pants hanging from her small frame were accented with oversized knits in a rainbow of blah, and the large and in charge power suits à la 1980 overwhelmed her petite figure. These suits in their bright primary colors screamed *Burn me*— and what a bonfire, in all its flammable nylon glory, that would be!

Ginny felt like she looked old, so she dressed even older. There were deeper issues underlying the fashion catastrophe that resulted from this approach. Aside from her gross misperceptions about her body—including "being soft," having "tons of gray," and looking "worn-out and drawn"—Ginny had misperceptions about who she was on the inside and who she thought she should be at age thirty-five.

Ginny felt that she should have been married, with children, that she should have bought her dream home, and that she should have landed her dream job. She felt great dissatisfaction with the timeline of her life. I assured her that this was a common feeling among women and men her age. Many people either don't feel that they are within the norm, as Ginny felt, or believe that they are trapped in the norm. Both are good reasons for dissatisfaction: a life should be in balance.

Because Ginny did not have a husband and children, she had time and freedom to travel, go to lectures, visit friends, and plan her days the way she pleased. The downside was the feeling that her window of opportunity to find a husband, have a child with him, and commit to a job search would soon be behind her. Ginny's wardrobe reflected her feeling that the exciting period of life was already over and merely a memory. To turn the clock back, Ginny needed to examine her internal fears, come up with an action plan, and create a wardrobe to match.

Healing Your Inner Ginny

As I did with Ginny, you can analyze your age from a full-life perspective and realize that you have much more of life to experience. Find biographies of people who found success and fulfillment late in their lives. For example, Grandma Moses didn't start drawing until she was in her seventies. Betty White successfully hosted *Saturday Night Live* when she was in her eighties.

Then ask yourself the three questions I asked Ginny: (1) If age were not a factor, what would you want to do? (2) What would you wish you had done when you're one hundred years old? (3) What would you like to tell your great-grandchildren about how you lived your life?

Thinking about these questions uninhibited by unreasonable age anxiety, you may find that your answers help you turn your desires into action. Ginny said that she will wish she had dated more, worried less, traveled more, gone back to school, and begun writing a book. So what did she do? She began *doing* it!

The next step is to come up with an action plan and life timeline, including due dates for specific goals. Ginny was able to break up her large goals into daily tasks that she wrote on a calendar.

Finally, work on the wardrobe. Life is short! There is no need to hasten the process, so why on earth would you dress older than you are? We've all seen the makeover shows featuring people who dress far older than they should and who seem to walk through life with an albatross around their neck. *Presto change-o*—after the makeover, all of them appear lighter, brighter, and younger. This transformation starts on the outside but fills the person on the inside.

Your clothes and accessories should facilitate the completion of your life goals. For each specific activity, find an outfit that you can wear while completing it. Ginny wanted to eventually get married, have children, and find a new job. We shopped for wardrobe basics in modern, form-fitting silhouettes, starting with underwear. I also eased her into saturated colors, which instantly brighten, not to mention draw the attention of others.

We have all heard that it is not the outcome but the process. It is not the destination but the journey. So what if Ginny did not get married or publish a book? At least she was working toward it.

Case Study: How Dressing Her Age Helped Frances Grow Up

I had spotted Frances as soon as I walked into the door at Starbucks, and my first thought was *Good Lord, this woman needs a makeover.* My second thought was, *And how old does this forty-something think she actually is?* Of course, I decided against going up to a stranger and saying, "Hey, I would loooove to make you over." Instead, I sat next to my friend to enjoy my mocha frappuccino.

Just as I was in the middle of telling my friend about InsideOut, my fashion psychology consulting business, Frances approached our table and introduced herself. One arm was stacked with neon jelly bracelets that resembled shapes of animals. She was swathed in a hot pink terrycloth jumpsuit with the words GIRL POWER stitched across the back in rhinestones. Her flip-flops, also hot pink, were adorned with charms. She was either actively resisting the aging process or passively clueless when it came to dressing for her age.

"Hi, I couldn't help overhearing about your idea," she said. "Could you please give me your email? I'm kinda in the midst of figuring out myself and my wardrobe, so I would love to possibly work with you in the future."

As if she had read my mind, Frances knew that she needed help. Her inside and outside were incongruent. We exchanged information and set up a consultation. In my office, we would quickly get to her core issues.

On the appointed day, Frances's arrival was announced by the clicking and clacking of her platform shearling clogs. The sweet smell of her glitter body spray and lip gloss was outdone only by her pleated plaid miniskirt, fitted cardigan, patterned tights, and, once again, the stack of jelly bracelets. Curled up on my therapeutic couch, Frances began telling her story.

"I've fought the aging process tooth and nail! Botox, lasers, acupuncture . . . you name it, I've done it." Frances could describe all of the anti-aging remedies in great detail, from cosmetic procedures in the West (Beverly Hills) to ancient healing rituals in the East (Vermont). But her age-defying ways had not stopped with procedures—they had leaked into every facet of her life, including her closet.

"Well, I know I am getting older, but I don't feel that way. I'm having a really hard time dressing my age without looking old, though, so instead I just try to dress younger. I don't think I am really doing that properly either."

"So where are you getting your style inspiration from now?"

"Well, I figure following my daughter and her style is my best bet to maintain freshness and currency. She is now seventeen. . . . Oh my gosh, I can't believe she is already seventeen!"

This remark was an indicator of an issue that went even deeper than trying to recapture her own youth—Frances was trying to capture her daughter's youth. She described how much she enjoyed shopping with her daughter and sharing clothes, habits she was going to miss when her daughter went off to college.

"Frances, you seem to mention your daughter quite frequently. It sounds like you two are very close?"

"Absolutely, we are each other's best friends."

After that admission, Frances and I threw all the items she brought from her closet on the couch to begin the purge. The main part of the initial process was to identify what worked, what didn't work, and, most importantly in each case, why. The second part of the process was to identify more *specifically* what it was about her aging experience that Frances was unable to manage.

"Okay, Frances, let's separate your clothes into two piles: what your daughter would wear, and what she wouldn't wear."

"Wait, don't you mean me?"

"No, definitely your daughter." This would now be an easier task for Frances. I imagined that if I had asked this question of her at the start, it would have taken much more time and effort. Sure enough, she quickly pulled out two-thirds of the clothes and designated them as appropriate for her daughter. What remained in the pile were clothes so dowdy that even my grandmother wouldn't have worn them.

"It looks like your piles reflect two states of being—the young and the old."

"Yeah, the pretty and the pretty ugly! I know, it's awful!"

Now for the obvious question. "What do you think *you* should wear from both piles?" I asked.

"That's the hardest. I really don't know. I'm having a really difficult time figuring out where I fit between the two categories."

"Well, Frances, quite frankly, I would say neither. You are an entirely new category that hasn't been considered yet. And that's our job—to find the new category."

We would do that the next day. For the moment, all we did was go through the clothes, examining them for stains, rips, and fit. Doing anything more than that would have thrown Frances into a panic— and right back to Forever 21!

Treatment

I visited Frances the next day at her house. "Frances," I asked, "when you were looking at your wardrobe yesterday, you acknowledged that it was split between juvenile and old lady. What's with that?"

"When I go to work or I need to be 'serious,' I pull out the old lady clothes, but all other times I want to feel young and hip, so I wear the cutesy clothes."

Somewhere in between serious and cutesy is where we were headed. I examined each piece in her wardrobe and wrote a list of possible replacements for the dowdy pieces.

Instead of:	Try:
Oversized silk blouse with a tie	Crisp French cuff shirt
Long wool pleated skirt	Knee-length panel-pleated skirt
Bulky turtlenecks	Soft cardigans and wraps

We would manage to replace the "serious" clothes in Frances's wardrobe with fresh and chic items. But the majority of her clothes should have been rocket-launched to her daughter's room. Still, Frances wanted to keep them.

"Why?" I asked her. "What do you feel would happen if we got rid of these?"

Eventually we got to the source. "I feel that if I give up those clothes, I give up the bond I have with my daughter, and I give up the part of me that was her age," Frances said. "I'm afraid we will lose this connection, and I will just be the old mom."

Frances went to great lengths to maintain the connection with her daughter, and this effort, she felt, required that she hold on to her own youth. She admitted trying to desperately keep up with her daughter by learning the lingo, the dress, the latest Perez Hilton gossip. This had seemed like the best strategy for staying close to her daughter.

But there was one major glitch in Frances's plan. When it came time for her to discipline her daughter, she was not taken seriously. Frances often let the rules and regulations slide. She had unconsciously decided that she could be the "best friend" and her husband could be the "mean parent."

To carry off the "young, hip, cool mom" routine, Frances had to adhere strictly to a wardrobe that matched. What began as a desire to simply maintain her physical appearance turned into a full regression; specifically, she swapped her maternal role for a friend role. If there is anything I know about parenting and development, children always need for their parents to be parents first before being friends.

Families require a hierarchy, which teaches children at the lower levels of the hierarchy that their parents or caretakers have things under control. When this hierarchy is in place, all the child has to worry about is being a child—trying hard in school, being kind to others, and so on. When a parent joins the child in being a child, there is no one to run the show. Often the child then feels unsecure or feels that he or she needs to step into the parental role. When children know who's in charge, the expectations, the rules of the game, and the consequences of poor behavior, they can relax into their role as a child and thrive.

Frances needed to see herself as an adult not only on the outside but on the inside. It was imperative that she begin to conceptualize herself as an effective adult parent who could maintain her "cool" without spiraling down into teenage-land. The first thing I had Frances do to establish that she was a forty-eight-year-old adult was to have her list behavioral guidelines for her daughter.

"Frances, it is time for you *and* your daughter to grow up. I want you to list all your daughter's behaviors that are disrespectful, inappropriate, or cross the line. After you list those behaviors, we are going to generate appropriate consequences for her."

After sitting for a while with a yellow legal pad, Frances started scribbling. Her list was quite extensive. We then worked on fine-tuning the consequences, and I gave her an assignment for the week: she was to sit with her daughter and tell her that there was a new sheriff in town, the sheriff had specific rules, and these rules were enforceable. Frances resisted the assignment, but I told her seek balance by making it a bad cop/good cop routine. In addition to laying down the law, Frances was to schedule some mother-daughter bonding time.

In a week's time I returned to see how she was managing her role as an *adult* mother. "Dr. B, it went surprisingly well. There was the initial shock of enforcing rules and some fighting, but overall it went pretty smoothly. My husband was completely surprised that I did what I did."

"Frances, you do not need to act like a teen to relate to one. You do not need to dress like a teen to feel young. That parenting exercise was to teach you how to do that. Just because you act like a mom doesn't mean you are destined to wear mommy jeans. Being an adult, an aging adult, is not something to be feared. Now, to the closet."

Reidentification

For a second time, I had Frances pull out the clothes that her daughter would wear, put them on, and look at herself in the mirror. When this exercise didn't have much of an impact on her, I took pictures of her in these outfits. Sometimes when you see yourself through an objective perspective you really see what you look like. This has happened to many of us: you wear an outfit you think is the most stylish getup in the world, and then two weeks later someone has posted pictures of you on Facebook and you are staring in horror at your outfit.

The pictures were key to giving Frances a chance to view herself with an objective eye. This forty-eight-year-old woman did not look young and hip in these clothes, and when she saw the pictures she realized that she looked like she was in costume for a high school play. Frances knew that she did not want to look old, but trying to look like a teen, she had to admit, was not working for her.

Modeling

If conceptualizing an "ideal look" is difficult for you, as it was for Frances, you can try copying a specific look to make it your own. Do you know a woman in your age range whose style you admire? And what about the plethora of successful, dynamic, and sophisticated women in the public eye these days? Whose style would you emulate?

Frances and I threw around many names—Oprah, Hillary Clinton, Raquel Welch, Laura Bush, Maya Angelou, and so on. When it came to the final vote, Jamie Lee Curtis won the election. She was to be Frances's role model for a healthy adult woman who was not afraid to embrace her age, her family, her body, and herself. When Frances felt unsure of how to handle a situation, from what to wear to how to handle her daughter, she would simply ask herself, *What would Jamie do?* After she decided on an answer, Frances would consider whether she felt comfortable doing what Jamie would do in that instance. This exercise helped Frances gain more and more confidence, and eventually she was directly asking herself: *What would Frances do?*

We put the final polish on Frances, working to make her external components—clothing, accessories, hair, makeup, speech—more grown-up. She had already looked through her clothes, thrown out the ripped and stained clothes, purged the "old lady stuff," seen herself looking ridiculous in the teenybopper wear, and was now ready to make the complete shift to a full-grown adult look. We pulled out a few of the go-to outfits in her wardrobe—the ones that she believed made her look "young and hip"—and I showed her how to make the adult version of them.

Not age-appropriate:	Age-appropriate:
Velour hot pink sweatsuit	Cashmere coordinates
Ripped jeans and bedazzled tank	Knee-length sequined sheath dress with peep-toe platform stilettos
Leggings and off-the-shoulder tunic with Ugg boots	Skinny jeans, riding boots, and a wrap cardigan

Frances's makeup went from neon and glitter to matte pastels. I threw out the scrunchies and ribbons, opting for sleek headbands and elastics.

Frances's return to her adult self took some trial and error and much refinement. As she became confident in her status as an adult, she lost interest in becoming younger and focused on getting older and better. She was no longer her daughter's "buddy," but a role model her daughter could be proud of. Now when Frances looked in the mirror, she didn't see a woman trying to be someone else, but the person she had grown up to become.

Helping Your Inner Frances

There is no doubt in my mind that people dress younger inappropriately because of fear . . . no, terror! Terror of getting older, terror of their mortality, terror of fading away. But the truth is that you can't hold on to the sands of time. The harder you grasp it the faster it slips out of your hands.

When it comes to assessing whether an article of clothing is "too young" to wear, just follow these shorthand guidelines:

If your daughter is wearing it, you should not.
If you have already worn a trend once, you should not wear it when it comes around again.
Just because you can fit into junior-size clothing does not mean you should rock it.

Avoiding anything your daughter would wear, not wearing the trend twice, and steering clear of the junior section may seem to address only your external appearance, but there is a significant internal component to these rules as well. If you aren't dressing age-appropriately, it might be time to question why. You want to "look cute" or "feel hot"? Dig deeper. The real reason could be:

I'm afraid I won't be noticed if I dress differently.
I'm afraid people will think I look old.
I'm afraid I will seem out of touch.
I'm unsure how to dress my age without looking frumpy.

Arrested Development

Besides halting the aging process, people often dress much younger than they should because they are stuck in an earlier time in their lives. You can stay forever young if you continue to shop in the juniors department, right? Wrong! It is common for people who have unresolved issues in their past to stay in that place to undo the wrong. For example, a woman who was teased in high school because she was "different" from the popular crowd may dress as an "in style" high schooler in adulthood. Conversely, if some point in the past was the zenith of your life, you may continue to dress in the style of that time even as you get older.

If you find yourself wearing clothing that is inappropriate for your age, you might want to consider *arrested development* as a possible explanation. Are you stuck in a certain period in your life? Was it the worst time of your life that you are trying to undo? Was it the high-light of your life that you are unwilling to give up?

To answer these questions, use old pictures or letters to put your-self back in this place and then examine what you are feeling there. To identify the root of the problem, you can use a Gestalt technique I use in therapy called the *empty chair*. In this session, I have patients imag-ine a loved one, a lost friend, or anyone with whom they have unfin-ished business. They speak to this person and imagine how he or she might respond, then they respond in turn to him or her. In this case, the empty chair can represent you in the past. Imagine your former self sitting there. You might need to tell that little girl who was teased that you are sorry it happened, you value her, things are different now, and she can let you move forward.

To get out of a period of arrested development, we need to move from the loss of the past while still honoring the experience. Truly moving away from our past can be difficult because we feel like a piece of ourselves has died. And we do indeed need to mourn that loss in order to move on and learn that we are still whole in the present.

Your Turn

The Energy of Clothes

When we talk about "dressing old," are we really referring to a certain age? I don't know about you, but I know many "old" ladies who are incredibly stylish. The first person who comes to mind is my grand-mother, who can be found wearing a leopard print three-quarter-sleeve swing coat and black beret . . . and she's ninety! God love her.

When we refer to a look as "old," it is not the measure of years that disturbs us—it is that, in our culture, "old" is associated with becoming irrelevant and unattractive. So when we say "old," more often than not what we are really trying to say is "out of style," "ugly," or "unflattering." Someone who is dressing "old" no longer cares what she looks like or what the rest of the world is wearing. She has given up!

We express our internal energies in our clothing choices. If you want to dress in a way that does not warrant the "old lady" descriptor, take age out of the equation and instead assess the level of energy your clothes emit. How do you do that? Just ask yourself these questions: How happy are you when you wear the garment? How many compliments do you receive? Does the garment improve your day or your performance? How attractive do you feel wearing it? The more energy there is in your clothes—the more alive you look and feel—the younger you appear to the outside world.

Quick Tips for Accepting the You in the Now

Identify who you are: Assessing your wardrobe periodically is an important part of maintaining self-awareness and reinventing yourself. Sadly, most people spend more time looking at the items they have in their closets than taking the time for self-inventory.

Much like a good closet cleaning, discovering what you have and what you need is essential for personal assessment. Purging the occasional bad item, such as a smoking habit or unhealthy dating pattern, is necessary to have the best life.

Accepting what you have to work with is also essential for a stylish wardrobe as well as a better you. No matter how much you wish it, you may never look good in camel. No matter how much you wish it; you may never have what it takes to become a sumo wrestler. No matter how much you wish it, you may never get any younger. You are where you are, you are who you are, and that is all that you are.

Identify who you want to be: Life is more exciting when you have room to expand. Desiring something better is the driving force for most lives. This is especially exciting when you try to amp up your wardrobe with pieces that refine your look. Your desire for something better shouldn't end with your closet. After examining who you are in your current life, make a plan for who you want to be and put it in writing.

Goal attainment keeps you young. It is only when you have nothing to live for that life is over, regardless of your age. There is always so much more to see and do! Who do you want to become?

Accept where you are: Yes, you have your fashion ideal. Yes, you have goals and dreams. Yes, you have a role model. Striving is healthy only when you are happy with the person you are now. If you feel less than that and are always hoping to be someone else, your efforts will fail. Even if you make both internal and external transformations, the change will come from an unhealthy place, the foundation will be unstable, and the new you will crumble.

It is only when you can accept who and where you are now in your life that you can consciously strive to become even better. The foundation for improvement is stable, and you love yourself so much that you are willing to give yourself the opportunity to enhance the already wonderful person you are.

Although you're a wonderful singer, you may decide to seek more training, study the vocal arts, work with other singers, or perform at public venues. Even when your clothes have wonderful style, you may want to work with the latest trends, push the envelope, or enter into the world of the avant-garde.

Plan to become who you want to be: You know who you are, and you have accepted it. You know what you want to be, and now it is time to put your plan into action and become it. A life without a plan is like a long road trip without a map. It is always good to know how to get to where you want to go; otherwise, you might drive right past your destination.

Make a plan and stick to it. You can make changes along the way, but a basic framework is essential. You can use this to create the wardrobe of your dreams, the job you have always wanted, or a friendship that will last a lifetime.

We have all heard that having a vision of what you desire helps you achieve. If you don't believe this, pick up a biography of an accomplished scientist, athlete, politician, or performer. Almost all of them had a dream. The second part of achievement is taking action to work toward your dream. The dream is the doorway, and the action is each brick in the pathway leading you to the front step.

Does the external match the internal? What if you know and love who you are, but look lousy? What if you have a plan for success, but don't take the time to look like it? If you have ever taken an acting class, performed onstage, or examined method actors, you know that looking the part is important when you are trying to get into character. It also helps the audience identify you as the character.

Your "costume" is your external appearance, which should match all that you are and all that you want to be. If you want a man to treat you properly, treat yourself properly. Take the time to comb your hair and wash your face. If you want the wonderful job, dress the part. Sweatpants don't make the cut. Even if you work at home, put on the nice dress. Trust me, it is just as comfortable. Want to retire to Florida? Then throw away your blacks and grays and start focusing on the whites, pinks, creams, oranges, and blues you will need when you move there. Let your clothing reflect your self-acceptance and self-love as well as propel you to achieve greater things.

Keeping It Fresh

Orient yourself: When creating the best and most updated wardrobe, you need to know who you are in the present. Go beyond your age and look at your daily activities, your size, your coloring, your budget, and your style preference. Your clothes should work with all of these components. Anything that does not work with who you are now should be given away or discarded. If you do not wear the item, if you feel uncomfortable when you wear it, or if you do not feel you're at your most attractive when wearing it, get rid of it.

Update your favorites: Everyone has specific items in their closet that they love, whether or not they're age-appropriate. Are you still wearing items you wore twenty years ago? Are you an older woman with items from the juniors section of the department store? Are you a younger woman with items from your grandmother's closet? If the answer is yes to any of these questions, it may be time to rework your favorites.

To get out of a style rut, identify the decade your item comes from and then find the current version of that item. If you want to maintain a vintage look, choose just one item from a past decade and make sure that the rest of your items are current. To make an outfit look younger, tighten the fit, shorten the length, use pastels and bright colors, mix prints, and multi-layer accessories. To make an item more mature, remove embellishments, keep a tailored cut, and stick to a neutral palette.

Avoid the "it" look: If your specific look defines a season, decade, celebrity, or collection, you have an "it" look. Although this look may work for a short period of time, it eventually becomes dated. To avoid this fashion trap, stick to the pieces that are "it" every season: a pair of straight-leg jeans, a dressy top, a trench, a ladylike sheath dress, and a killer heel. Although they may change slightly every two to five years, the general bones of these pieces remain.

Learn from your peers: Look around you. What are most women your age wearing? Whose style do you admire? When you watch TV or browse the Internet, what is worn by the women who are deemed stylish, sophisticated . . . and age-appropriate? What is their formula? Sleek and simple? Colorful and embellished? Classic or modern? Vintage or trendy? Long and loose? Fit and flare? Complicated clothes with simple accessories? Clean items with statement accents? They have done the work for you; just follow the formula.

Your age does not measure anything more than the time you have had on this earth. To give this number any more importance than that is a waste of time. Your age in no way indicates your ability, relevance, worth, importance, or impact. Don't push your age forward, don't hold it back, and don't get stuck in it.

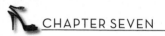

CHAPTER SEVEN

Working for It

When You Find Yourself Forever in Work Clothes

Our "work history" does not begin with the first day of our first job. Striving for occupational greatness begins at a very young age, as soon as we start taking tests and exams that assess our intellectual performance. Our paths have often been laid out for us by the time we learn to walk. These days, prepping for kindergarten can include learning multiple languages, music classes, and athletic pursuits!

As a psychologist, I often become part of the "achievement process" by providing cognitive assessments, which measure factors such as a child's intelligence, working memory, information processing, attention, and academic achievement. These assessments are requested to examine any difficulties a child might have that would impair learning, specifically school performance. Yet it is through cognitive assessments of a child that I often learn the most about the parents' aspirations for their child.

After at least two full days of observing, interviewing, and testing and a week of scoring, interpreting, and integrating, I'm ready to deliver a full cognitive report. The parents and children are then called to discuss the findings. This day is full of anticipation and anxiety, as accommodations and admissions are often riding on the results. After assuring the parents that their child is "within an average range," I am always shocked at their dissatisfaction with statistical normalcy. Deeper examination has often revealed that their feelings are not a response to the scores, but to the associations they attach to the scores. They believe that these scores are directly correlated to their child's eventual academic and vocational success.

Many of us dedicate anywhere from twelve to twenty years of our lives—from the time of early tests in elementary school to the moment when we gain acceptance to a prestigious university and graduate school—working to achieve the ultimate prize. All our academic struggles, networking efforts, unpaid internships, summer jobs, interviews, rejections, and after-school activities, as well as our parents' hopes and dreams for us, culminate in landing a good job.

But the incessant measuring does not end here. After we stop measuring our academic achievements, we'll turn to measuring our career achievements. Now we may discover that it's impossible to extract ourselves from our work after the nine-to-five shift is over. Many of us then extend our hours to include overtime and weekends. Our work leaks into our home, facilitated by business phones in our bedrooms and computers in our family rooms. On vacation we pack the BlackBerry, and if we are going home sick, we don't forget to bring the laptop with us. It's no wonder that our conceptualization of our identity is often lost to our work!

A Working Wardrobe

Our attitudes about our work life can change what we wear and how we wear it. Our mistakes can include both dressing inappropriately for the workplace and wearing only work clothes all the time, even outside of the office. Both mistakes indicate an inability to draw clear boundaries between work life and other life.

Looking the Part at the Office

Some people look like they're not even employed; they think it's acceptable to arrive in the workplace looking like they're lounging in their bedroom. These people just can't be bothered with the "frivolity" of apparel.

When it comes to your job, however, looking the part is important. In the workplace, people initially measure your level of professionalism by your appearance, and this first impression almost always sticks. When you don't take the time to dress professionally, your appearance detracts from the rest of you. If you were in a session with me and noticed a piece of toilet paper dragging along the bottom of my shoe, you would focus on that and become distracted from the session. It works the same way if I wear torn-up jeans and a sweat-stained shirt—you become fixated on my clothes and not on my work.

So what does "looking the part" mean? Gather clues from your environment. Where are you in the world? Are you in southern California, where casual is acceptable? Or are you in London, where a suit might be in order? Each region of the world has a way of dressing. Know your style latitude and longitude.

Begin to narrow the focus from your country and region to your workplace. What kind of environment do you work in? Are most people dressed casually or formally? Is it all work or play? Is the look stratified? For example, are the higher-ups wearing the suits while the worker bees wear leggings and tunics?

Dressing for the country, region, and workplace are important, but dressing for your customer—the person you are selling your product to, whether it is hamburgers or therapy—should be your top priority. It's your customers who keep you in business, provide recommendations, refer future customers, give testimonials, and call your boss with glowing reports. Give the customer what he or she wants through your wardrobe as well as your work ethic. Every consultation class or public speaking training stresses the need to know your audience. One important way to know your audience is to know what they'd like for you to wear to create a connection and make them confident that you are the ultimate person for the job.

When I first began my job on the West Coast, I brought along my East Coast work outfits: suits, sheath dresses, heels, jewelry, trenches, and so on. My workplace, however, turned out to be very casual: the only time employees dressed up was for all-staff presentations, and the one wearing the suit was the presenter. I was encouraged to dress down because I was told that patients could not relate to me if I dressed formally.

Yet the patients actually said quite the opposite. They appreciated that I valued them enough to dress up for my job and serve them. Many of them who felt worn down by life and the "system" were appreciative that I thought they were "worth it." I wanted to look nice for them because I valued and respected them.

You also need to think about what you are doing with your audience. Are you sitting at a desk with them in air-conditioned comfort? Or are you walking across town in the sweltering heat? To make your client feel comfortable, you must look like you can effortlessly execute your job duties. Hobbling in four-inch heels with your feet covered in blisters does not translate into competence.

Maybe you are afraid to dress well because you think people may not take you seriously. For women, gender issues often contribute to this fear. Can we dress well and still be perceived as having a fully functioning frontal lobe? Is it only when we sacrifice our taste that we can be taken seriously? Must we wear dull shoes and synthetic fiber suits to feel professional?

I understand the working woman's struggle because I have lived it. Like many of you, I have felt that in order to be perceived as professional and intelligent, I had to tone myself down or look like I didn't care too much about my appearance. The struggle is to find our style in an intelligent way. Anyone who does not take us seriously because we take dress as seriously as we do any other skill is most likely grappling with their own insecurities.

If you are in school or in the workforce, dress for the position you desire. If you are a secretary and want to be head of the company, dress like the head of the company. If you are a student and want to become the professor, dress like one. The people who make the snippy comments are not the ones who are going to promote you. Remember: as we climb up the ladder, only the most stylish of stilettos can handle the pressure!

Anyone can look like a well-dressed employee. But with hard work, dedication, and the talent to back up a hot wardrobe, your beautiful look can serve to package an exceptional product. Gives whole new meaning to the phrase "work it!"

Are You Working Too Much? A Checklist

For every employee who does not dress professionally on the job, there is one who dresses for her job even on the off days. This individual is so consumed with her life at the workplace that she forgets about other areas of her life. Sadly, the closet is filled with professional attire, leaving no time or room for anything else. Sound familiar?

❏ When you are not at work, do you think about it often?

❏ Do you have trouble sleeping because you are thinking about all the work you have to do the next morning?

❏ During your days off, do you have trouble relaxing?

❏ Are you glued to your mobile devices when you are not at work?

❏ Do you find vacations more difficult because they ultimately create more work upon your return?

❏ Do you go to work on the weekends?

❏ Do you skip breaks and lunch to continue working?

❏ Are your only friends your work colleagues?

❏ Do you find that when you are not at work you have nothing to do?

❏ Have your friends and family expressed concern about your work habits?

❏ Do you want a better work-life balance but don't know how to achieve it?

❏ Have you experienced mental or physical exhaustion because of work?

❏ When you are not working, do you wear work clothes?

❏ When you have to dress for a nonwork function, do you have anything other than work attire to wear?

❏ Have you shopped within the last year for nonwork clothes? Within the past six months?

❏ When shopping for nonwork clothes, are you unsure of what to buy?

❏ Do you want to make changes in your wardrobe but don't know how to do it?

If you answered yes to most of these questions, you may be a workaholic. Your new job: achieving a work-life balance and crafting a wardrobe to match!

THE DOS AND DON'TS OF OFFICE WEAR

Quality

Don't wear clothes with broken closures.
Do find a good seamstress or conceal closures with a
    stylish belt or pin.

Don't wear clothes with holes in them.
Do invest in a sewing kit or a trash can!

Don't wear clothing with lint, dog hair, or pills on it.
Do invest in a lint remover, a plastic depilling comb, or a
    sweater shaver.

Don't wear stained garments.
Do buy an on-the-go stain remover and fabric sweat guards.

Fit

Don't wear anything too tight, too short, or too loose.
Do make an appointment with a personal shopper to learn
    how to find clothes that fit properly.

Don't display your visible panty line (VPL).
Do bring your clothes when you shop in the lingerie
    department so that you can find the perfect undergarments
    for each outfit.

Don't expose your breast or posterior cleavage.
Do make sure that you can lean, bend, sit, and stand
    without exposure.

continues

THE DOES AND DON'TS OF OFFICE WEAR   *continued*

Function

Don't wear uncomfortable, wobbly, or blister-inducing shoes.
Do buy high heels a half-size larger for comfort, and invest
    in gel inserts.

Don't wear clothes that inhibit you from doing your job.
Do wear stylish clothes that are breathable and allow
    movement.

Don't become a victim of air conditioning or heat.
Do buy pieces you can peel off and layer on.

Style

Don't engage on theme dressing (nautical, safari, punk,
    and so on).
Do choose one piece from your favorite theme to mix with
    classic items.

Don't ostracize yourself with your style choices.
Do follow the climate of the workplace dress (conservative,
    trendy, formal, casual, and so on).

Don't dress exactly like everyone else.
Do lend personality to your look by adding your own favorite
    style touches.

Don't wear accessories that make too much noise.
Do add a small rubber heel cover on your shoes and swap the
    jingly bangles for cuffs.

Don't wear offensive messages on your clothing.
Do consider how your words, even on clothes, affect others.

Case Study: Why Looking the Part
Was Part of Megan's Job

Megan, a physician, lived in her scrubs. Both in and out of the hospital, she wore heart-and-puppy-dog-print smocks with white rubber clogs everywhere and anywhere. Megan worked in her scrubs, relaxed in her scrubs, did errands in her scrubs, and even slept in her scrubs. When it came to taking this part of her wardrobe as far as it could go, Megan stretched the limits. She may have been an expert in medicine, but when it came to her wardrobe she was flatlining.

One weekend Megan realized that she had hit fashion rock bottom. She called me in desperation. This was one emergency that Megan was not able to handle in her health care *habillements*.

"Dr. B, I have totally embarrassed myself. I ran into my coworker this weekend, and I was still wearing my work clothes. Oh God, he must think that I don't shower, or have a life for that matter. What a nightmare."

Megan's distress reminded me of when my own work life threatened to overwhelm my regular life: I spent the first half of my academic career almost exclusively in kilts and polos. I was ready to help Megan find her real-life wardrobe, as I had found mine so long ago. It was time to go to the primary source of Megan's image ailment—her closet.

When I arrived at her apartment, Megan said, "Okay, it's so pathetic to admit this, but outside of work clothes, I literally have nothing to wear. I mean, I have stuff—I am just not sure what to do with it. What is even more pathetic is that I would not have even noticed this if my hot freakin' coworker hadn't asked me if I was on call this weekend. Yeah, aaahhh, no, I wasn't."

"So basically, Megan, your wardrobe has no life, and our job is to get it one," I said. What I didn't say was, *And we will get you one as well*.

Why was it that she could put on a work outfit but couldn't pull together a Sunday grocery shopping ensemble or a date look? Megan liked the ease of always wearing a uniform. Scrubs and clogs were interchangeable and required little thought . . . or effort!

Unfortunately, her current wardrobe made her look like an extra on *ER*. We would need to acknowledge her preference for a "uniform" wardrobe by creating a similar ease of dress for her nonwork wear. As a young physician starting a practice and still paying off her student loans, Megan was also on a limited income. She wanted reasonably priced pieces that could be used for multiple functions. Her new wardrobe pieces needed to fit into various areas of her life without blowing her budget. Finally, Megan needed clothes that were comfortable. Her activities outside of work included traveling, walking, lounging, and casual outings, and she wanted to be free to move around comfortably and navigate her day without the constriction of binding clothes and inflexible shoes.

The answer to Megan's woes was *capsule dressing,* a no-brainer wardrobe built only on essential interchangeable pieces. Taking the coordinates, multi-functionality, and comfort of her current wardrobe and translating those qualities into a new wardrobe would be our primary goal for Megan's external makeover.

We had a clear shopping plan before we even looked at her closet, and I was confident that her transition from Dr. Megan to Megan would be a smooth one. But when we opened the bedroom closet, I was unable to find any "normal" clothing. Each hanger held only doctor gear. I asked Megan to show me the rest of her wardrobe.

Megan flushed. "Uhhh, do you really want to know?" she asked. I nodded my head. "Well, they are in the laundry room." I raised my eyebrows, and Megan led me to the laundry room, also known in her case as "the second closet." Dirty clothes covered the concrete floor, washed clothes were still in baskets, and a dryer that hadn't been started was stuffed with wet jeans.

"Megan, I see a bunch of clothes stuck in laundry limbo. When's the last time you've ever worn this stuff? We need to gather all of your clothes into one area of the house so that I can see what you are working with."

Megan stared off into the distance. "Well, to be quite honest, I really haven't had time to wear most of this stuff lately. The only thing that I really get to wear are the scrubs upstairs."

After completing a cycle in the dryer, Megan and I collected all of the clothes and carted them up to her room. The first part of the makeover process was to examine her lifestyle to find categories of dress. I had Megan separate her clothing into categories, which included casual weekend, night out, formal events, workout gear, and pajamas. As Megan cursed under her breath and jumped back and forth among the random piles, I realized that she could not fill these categories from the pieces we had in front of us. Upon deeper examination, I realized that these clothes dated from her pre–medical school days. Megan had not shopped in so long that she could not wear what she had. Hardly anything fit or was in style.

"Megan, my friend, I see why you can't make anything from this wardrobe. The only clothes you have that can be worn are your work clothes. Now I know why you only wear them and nothing else."

Being a surgeon's daughter, I knew all about the time commitment that doctors make to their calling. My father had to work just as hard balancing his work life and home life as he did getting into medical school. The burden of improving patients' health can wreak havoc on a physician's personal life. Megan's wardrobe situation was a clear indication that she was consumed by her job. There was no room in her life or closet for anything else. But Megan's obligations needed to include herself before she lost herself to work entirely.

"What is your schedule like during the week?" I asked. "How much time are you dedicating to your job, and how much time are you dedicating to the rest of your life?"

As I worked through this process with her, Megan realized that her life was fully saturated with work. She had been on the job treadmill for so long that she never realized that she rarely took time for her own needs. When she was not working, Megan was not engaged in any activity. A life this unbalanced was no life at all, and Megan needed a far greater change than the one to her wardrobe.

Treatment

Before I left her house, I asked Megan to friend me on Facebook. I wanted to begin my investigation of who Megan thought she was, and online social networks are a great way to gather clues. It is not *what* we say to others but *how* we present ourselves that gives them the greatest insight into us. Just as I suspected, Megan's profile read like a résumé. All of her accomplishments and affiliations were posted. Every picture was clearly a catalog of a success. There is absolutely nothing wrong with being proud of yourself, but Megan was merely a compilation of external evaluations. Without those, Megan could not see her own worth.

Self-inspection is useless without action. Megan's awareness of the imbalance in her life would not be productive if I did not push her toward active change.

The next session I arrived early at Megan's house and asked her to write down words that described herself. All of her descriptors pointed to external accomplishments—titles, awards, degrees. Besides "doctor, top of my class, Ivy League grad," Megan could not think of any internal qualities to describe herself. She had lost herself among her accomplishments.

"Where is Megan in all of this?" She looked at me like I had lost my mind. I repeated the question.

"This is me, this is who I am. I am not quite sure what you are looking for."

"Megan, I am sure there is more to you than this. I see nothing here but a résumé. I would like to see the things that make you uniquely you. There is nothing wrong with pride in your academic and medical achievements, but I believe this has become your identity. Try the exercise again, but this time I want you to write about Megan without the résumé builders."

Megan agreed to try describing herself this way, but this time the task took far longer. For years she had spent so much time and energy with her eyes on the prize. When she achieved the prize, she set up another. First, it had been getting into a fantastic college, then it was getting into medical school, and now it was building a private practice.

"Okay, here it is. I've got my list, but it was so hard to write. I kept resisting the urge to write a résumé. Here it is: giver, empathic, and analytic."

"That's great, Megan. This is what I'm talking about. Now let's see if we can make this a habit."

Megan liked having a plan of action, so I gave her one. I wanted her to turn inward rather than outward to learn who she was. She was used to gathering external input to measure her inner value. But external validation is always a recipe for disaster: it counts for only so much before it deflates you.

Megan had her assignment: to fill her social calendar with events involving others who were not in the medical sciences. She needed to spend time in a new world with new people who were not affiliated with her profession.

Megan's second task was a prohibition. She was forbidden for a month to speak of any of her accomplishments when she met someone new during her social adventures. I taught her all the tricks of *deflection* that psychologists are trained to use when clients ask us personal questions.

"Megan, it's time to learn Clinical Interviewing 101. When someone asks what you studied, tell them you are a student of life, you had a liberal arts education, or you enjoyed all areas of study. Then immediately turn the conversation back to them with a question about their course of study, a question directed at an internal quality, or a question you would like them to eventually ask you."

As I taught Megan how to avoid answering the profession questions, we generated some responses and possible deflectors. "So if someone asks me what I do, I am going to tell them I have dedicated my life to helping people. If they continue to ask, I am going to say that I work as a scientist or in medical sciences. Then I am going to ask them what they do, or change the subject, or even talk about something that I take pride in."

Megan went out and pursued activities and social events that brought passion to her life rather than another checklist, taking with her what she had learned about focusing on her internal accomplishments and interests as well as these aspects of others. After a month of this exercise, I revisited Megan and her closet.

"Okay, Megan, how was it?"

"Resisting the urge to tell people what I do and where I went to school required a concentrated effort. I realized how much saying those things gives me a false importance. Without it, I was left with no other option but to question what really makes me important and special. Would my existence be worthwhile if I had not accomplished those things?"

"So what was the answer?"

"I actually learned the answer by asking others about their lives. You always hear that we have inherent worth when we arrive in this world, and you fully believe it about others, but to fully believe that about yourself? That is almost impossible."

Megan had to learn that her value judgments about other people, which focused on their internal qualities and inherent worth, were applicable to herself as well. Why was it that others could fail at school, not go to school, or have a job with no title and still be something, but she couldn't? It was through this exercise that Megan finally realized her worth.

Megan also needed to add downtime to her busy life. To help her find her work-life balance, I told Megan to schedule time to simply do nothing. We dusted off her day planner. Megan worked full days on Monday, Tuesday, and Thursday. After these long days, Megan scheduled "relaxation time" at night. Her idea of doing nothing was catching up with her favorite shows, which included *Oprah's Lifeclass* and reruns of *RuPaul's Drag Race*. On her half-days, Wednesday and Friday, Megan was excited to make plans with friends, play kickball, and explore her neighborhood's culinary offerings. Saturday and Sunday were the days for adventure and excitement—anything from a road trip to a blind date.

Reidentification

"You really know who you are now," I told Megan. "You know who you are with or without your external accomplishments. After releasing those parts that you thought were so essential to your identity, you found your true identity."

Megan now felt free to pursue activities that in the past she would have deemed "professionally inappropriate." Through her interactions with others, she realized how worthwhile it was to do something for no other purpose than to have fun. Megan learned to find joy in joining a kickball team and continuing to dance without the purpose of competing, and speed-dating (she was still, after all, a busy doctor).

The final step in Megan's InsideOut makeover was to find the new wardrobe that would match her new identity. When you know who you are . . . really know who you are . . . dressing becomes very easy. Megan was a doctor, but she was also an intelligent go-getter. She felt best in clothes that reflected all that she felt inside. She still wanted comfortable and affordable clothing, so we turned to sharply tailored classics with low kitten heels to make her feel everything that she was. On the weekends she felt that she was an adventurer and an explorer, always hungry for the next new thing. We looked for clothing full of bright color and spice, just like the food she loved. These clothes were less structured than her work clothes. She enjoyed Indian-inspired clothing and jewelry, so she selected bright tunics to wear with a gold bangle or hoop. These items were easily found at Zara and H&M. When you know what looks good, and good on you, you really can shop anywhere at any price point and look divine.

One month later, Megan greeted me at her door wearing wedge heels with a flouncy patterned skirt and a bright tank top. She was getting ready for a date with a coworker, whom she had never noticed until she took the time and made the effort to sit in the break room for lunch.

"I feel totally in balance. I can relax from my job and the identity of being a doctor. During the night and weekend, I can just be Megan. And when I feel a little bored with being Megan, I'm back to being Dr. Megan." Megan didn't lose the part of her identity for which she had worked so hard—being a doctor—but did fill in the missing pieces of her life. Standing before me was a three-dimensional Megan, a whole person. And as much as I was tempted to ask her about the best medical remedy for dark circles under the eyes, I resisted. Megan was off the clock!

Your Turn

Lose the Job

Like Megan, many of us attach a great deal of our time, identity, and worth to our job. Most introductory conversations with others include the question "What do you do?" And when we're not discussing work we talk about our hobbies, charitable deeds, social endeavors, and other accomplishments.

With technological advances, our hours on the job are no longer limited to the office. What was originally intended to make our jobs easier, however, has actually created more work for us during our private time. Our work life seeps into our personal life, and often our external world reflects that shift. Homes are no longer homes—they are work outposts, or even headquarters. Bedrooms serve as catchalls for files, important paperwork, and unfinished business. Our cars have become mobile storage units for work shoes, changes of clothing, and snacks. Even our wardrobes may reflect nothing but work, work, work. Where is the "you" in this scenario?

I struggled with life-work balance while in graduate school. Most of my time, energy, identity, and understanding of success was pinned on my work. I had so little time for anything besides reading, writing, studying, preparing, applying, diagnosing, and treating that all the other parts of me disappeared. When I finally had a break to go out with my friends or on a date, I literally had nothing to wear! During the period between graduation and post-licensure employment, my entire wardrobe consisted of suit pants, fancy sweaters, button-downs, pencil skirts, blazers, and heels. I needed to go shopping, but unfortunately, shopping did not solve my greater problem. I was so accustomed to living for work that when I was working there was nothing else going on in my life, and when I wasn't working my life lost its meaning.

If you are like Megan and me, struggling with your identity and purpose outside of work, try approaching this "search for self" in steps, as you would a job search.

1. *List the activities you love:* For instance, maybe you like to read, shop, cook, or give advice to others.

2. *Find an activity in which you can find success:* Are you an excellent runner, painter, or singer? In examining your hobbies, don't measure success by the end result. If you can reasonably accomplish what's needed to enjoy an activity, then you are successful. More than likely, your list of activities you engage in during your free time overlaps considerably with your list of activities you can perform successfully.

3. *Circle the top five activities that you can reasonably accomplish:* Do not, however, make this yet another work task.

4. *Go with it!* Start pursing the top activity on your list with a reasonable plan and due date. If, after much pursuit, the activity is no longer pleasurable or impossible to be successful at, rework it or go to the second one on your list.

Now you are no longer just a worker bee—you are an actor, singer, writer, painter, advocate, healer, or mentor. When I tried this exercise, my top activities were in being engaged in fashion pursuits, helping others, educating the public about wellness, and writing. And what happened as a result of that simple exercise? You're reading it!

Many of us cannot separate ourselves and our wardrobes from our work. Therefore, we must learn to lose our job when we are not at work.

Quick Tips for
Finding the Work-Life Balance

Examine and identify: If you don't look for a problem, you may not find one. Are you one of those people so busy working that they don't have the time to examine their life? Even if you haven't noticed, someone else probably has noted that your scales are off balance. You need to work less and play more.

Growth requires self-examination. Take the time and energy to look at your calendar—yearly, monthly, weekly, or daily. Do you find that the pie chart of your life is consumed by your job? If the answer is yes, make it your job to replace work with something else. Wishing that your life would become balanced will not change it, and getting someone else to help you find balance will not change it. You yourself must take *action* to balance your life. Without a conscious change in behavior, your life will remain the same.

Regroup and reschedule: If you have made the effort to examine your life and come to the realization that it is out of balance, you must change your daily patterns to balance the scales. I know that we all have busy schedules and that technological advances have made work a part of our nonwork lives, but you still must draw the line in the sand. Balancing requires boundaries.

We have boundaries for most elements of our lives: friendships, family members, foods, physical activities, and so on. You must build boundaries to contain your work. Start by placing *temporal* limits on the amount of time you take out of your day to be at work and produce work. For example, try restricting the time you spend working on weekends to the early morning hours only. Impose *physical* boundaries by separating your home space and your work space and maintain these boundaries by eliminating work materials, such as computers, papers, projects, or files, from your bedroom.

Drawing *mental* boundaries requires becoming aware of your thoughts, words, and actions that are work-focused versus those that are not. Stopping your thoughts about work when you are relaxing with your family is a way of drawing a mental boundary. Finally, you must put *emotional* boundaries, which are the most difficult to draw, on your work. Emotional boundaries include anything that moves you internally. For example, relieving your anxiety about work through practicing meditation is one of many ways to create such boundaries.

Take what you can get and steal moments: Even during the most difficult days there are small slivers of time that are yours alone. The moments in your bed right before you need to leave it, the time while you're dressing, the instant you sip your coffee, the pause to freshen up in the bathroom, your walk to the office, the lull between clients, the ride home, and the quiet space between going to bed and going to sleep. Although limited in number and short in duration, these moments do exist, and they are yours for the taking. Do not let them slip by unnoticed. Use them as a break from your workday. See them as a deposit in an energy bank that may be approaching depletion.

Use other small opportunities to balance your day. Making your work space beautiful with fresh flowers, a beautiful picture, a nice pillow, or some soft music can make you feel in balance. Make your ordinary daily routines extraordinary. Don't eat at your desk when you can take your meal outside instead. Bring a gourmet lunch from home rather than eating cafeteria food. Try dressing for work as if you were dressing for a wonderful outing. Seeing the best version of yourself reflected off your computer screen can add brightness to the darkest of workdays.

Minimize and compartmentalize: Put your work obligations and stressors into perspective. Does the project you're stressing over really warrant this investment of high emotion? Will you care about it in a week, a month, or a year? Probably not. Do what you actually need to do and nothing more if your life feels supersaturated with work. Any precious time you spend on work that should be used for relaxation, socialization, and hobbies instead is a waste of time. Work more efficiently, not more. If you remove distractions during work hours, you can get as much done in half the time and then have even more time for leisure.

Learn to leave work at work. Many people ask me whether I take my patients home with me, whether I keep thinking about them, especially those who have horrible life circumstances, after I leave my office. I always tell them that I would not be able to do my job effectively if I did. How can I work well at work if I'm still working at home in my head? When you are at your job, be present 100 percent. When you leave, do not track work home on the bottoms of your shoes!

Support and surrender: Sometimes there's nothing better than turning to the crew of your ship during a long and laborious voyage. If you are all in the same boat, find the time to commiserate, brainstorm, and support each other. Just when you feel that you can't take any more, a smile or a joke may make it all better.

Finding balance when you're overloaded at work requires that you decrease your work per person or add another person. There is no shame in asking someone to help you. Surrendering to your limitations is one of the primary obligations of a balanced life.

Capsule Dressing 101

If you are short on time and energy, *capsule dressing* is the best option for crafting a wardrobe. This method uses the least number of pieces to create the greatest number of looks. Think back to a grade school word problem: given a list of words, you were told to calculate the number of possible word combinations from that list. The outcome was a very large number based on the exponential growth of your combinations. The capsule method of dressing offers the same numerical outcome—many outfits.

Donna Karan popularized capsule dressing in the 1980s with her capsule collection, which offered "seven easy pieces"—a bodysuit, a coat, a jacket, a blouse, a skirt, pants, and a dress for evening. Since then, other designers have introduced capsule collections for busy working women, women on a budget, or women who need help crafting a wardrobe.

But you don't need a designer to create your own capsule collection. Begin by choosing five to fifteen pieces you can wear anytime, anyplace. If you were about to be stranded on a desert island, or your house were on fire, what items would you take with you to have a functional wardrobe? For example, one sheath dress, a blazer, leggings, and a top.

Make sure all the pieces you choose can mix and match. For example, make all of your pieces either cream or black. Remove any piece that is unnecessary or has a function that could be accomplished with another piece. For example, I don't need leggings when I have pants that serve the same function. Finally, accessorize: wear riding boots, high boots, ankle booties, pumps, wedges, strappy heels, tights, sheer stockings, jewelry, scarves, and hats.

Remember: the purpose of the capsule collection is to have an efficient wardrobe with the least number of items. There is no room for extras with this method. You should be able to pack your entire collection into a small suitcase and have a fully functional wardrobe. If crafting a capsule wardrobe is difficult for you, be sure to read

Nina Garcia's *The One Hundred: A Guide to the Pieces Every Stylish Woman Must Own.** In this book she lists one hundred essential pieces that you can choose from to create a minimal wardrobe with maximum impact.

For most of us, work is not a choice but a necessity. Whether we despise our jobs or find joy in them, the tendency to overwork is a difficult temptation to resist. Nevertheless, living to work is not a life. If you are spending the majority of your existence working, you do not truly exist. But you can make it your job to bring about changes that will restore balance to your life and, in those areas of your job that you can control, infuse some joy into your day.

---

* N. Garcia, *The One Hundred: A Guide to the Pieces Every Stylish Woman Must Own* (New York: HarperCollins, 2008).

CHAPTER EIGHT

It's All in the Details

When You Are Covered in Labels

In fashion, *who* you are wearing is an opportunity to advertise who you are. Articles of clothing—shirts, scarves, dresses—are neutral stimuli; they have no inherent capacity to generate a response from us. We learn to associate meaning with these items through *classical conditioning*. What brand advertisers do is pair neutral stimuli with provocative images that do elicit a response. Eventually, we respond to brands even in the absence of the original stimulus.

For example, imagine walking into an Abercrombie store and staring into the eyes of a hot naked man on a horse. This stimulus elicits an emotional response of . . . oh, I don't know . . . let's say *lust!* Eventually, you associate Abercrombie clothing with sexiness. Eventually you don't even need pictures of naked models in compromising positions to equate Abercrombie with sexiness— just seeing the label or the name is enough. Abercrombie hopes that you will want to feel sexy and will want others to associate you with sexiness, and so will buy its clothing.

Designers and advertisers depend on and profit from our emotional experiences with our clothing and our desire to elicit the same emotional experiences from others. When you buy designer clothing, you are no longer buying mere pieces of fabric—you are buying everything associated with the brand. You are buying into the "feel" of the brand experience. And in turn, you are buying the opportunity to convey that this brand represents a part of you.

So how is the "feel" created? Advertisements, whether in the glossy pages of *Town and Country* or flashing onto our plasma screens, feature the brand, not the product, as the central part of the experience. If advertisers have done their job, we feel something after viewing these ads: aroused, relaxed, joyful, invigorated.

Another technique is to use a representative for the brand, which can be a person, place, or thing. A movie star, dripping with pearls and sequins, at the Eiffel Tower. A polo field in Spain dotted with thoroughbreds and sun hats. A white Rolls-Royce with cashmere blankets and caramel suede driving gloves on monogrammed leather seats. The psychology of social influence tells us that it is members of our *reference group*—which often includes people we admire who are featured in advertisements—who persuade us to buy their belongings.

These forms of enticement do not stop with the advertisements, but continue throughout the store. The music, the lights, the flowers, the champagne. What was once a room filled with shelving and racks of clothing has now been converted into a posh dressing salon. These items are used to enhance not only the shopping experience, so that you will stay longer and buy, but the brand identity. These atmospheric and decorative elements—the soundtrack, the level of illumination, the room temperature, and the décor—are not randomly chosen but carefully selected by a highly trained staff. Nothing is left to chance.

Even the people working in the stores are simply an extension of the brand. From my retail experience with both high- and low-end stores, I can tell you that every detail—from the greetings I used to answer the phone to the color of my nail polish—was carefully monitored. In one store, I was not allowed to wear black clothing or jewelry of any kind, and I was encouraged to ignore the customers unless spoken to. At another store, I was told to always "look busy" on the floor so that customers would believe that merchandise was "going fast." At yet another store, I spent a day learning nothing but how to package the purchase, give the purchase to the customer, and return the method of payment.

The store and its employees become part of the selling point, part of the brand. The unspoken words resounding from sales associates are: *If you buy our clothes, this experience can be yours too.*

Tell Me About Yourself

We become our own billboards, sometimes literally. From the sublime to the ridiculous, statements on your clothing send clear messages. You think BOYS ARE CUTE, and you support St. Jude's Children's Hospital. You tell the world that I VOTED TODAY or I KISS COWBOYS. Perhaps you ran the TURKEY TROT 2000 or play COED NAKED LACROSSE. Everyone who sees you learns that you were the president of the debate club at SQUIRREL TOOTH UNIVERSITY and that while you were there you pledged DELTA DELTA DELTA. These messages are bumper stickers for the body. The world gets a glimpse of your interests, likes, dislikes, causes, and activities.

Okay, I'll admit it—I was once obsessed with the message T-shirt. And I am not talking about marathons or nonprofits, I am talking about I HEART SKINNY BOYS WITH GLASSES and GET YOUR HOT BUNS IN HERE BAKERY.

Whether the message is from stamped tees or designer names, examining why you have chosen to tell the world about yourself in this way can lead to fruitful self-analysis. Do you wear these items just because you like them? Do you wear them because you're insecure in who you are without them? Do you wear them because you're trying to hide behind them? Do you wear them hoping to spark conversation? Do you wear them to tell the world of your accomplishments?

The Logo

Advertisements are certainly not limited to television, magazines, and storefronts. You, the customer, become the walking talking billboard for the brand you love when you wear its logo. Have you ever seen the guy dressed in a banana suit dancing along a main road enticing you to come into his store for a closer look? Well, guess what? You are that guy.

Logos are incredibly powerful symbols that companies use in order to sell their products and acquire loyal clientele. Whether it is the iconic Burberry plaid or the interlocking C's of Chanel, logos become the watermark for a certain standard of living as established by the brand. If we wear logos, we are saying that we support the label as well as the lifestyle that goes along with it. Logos are especially effective when used to establish a status hierarchy. The message of these logos is loud and clear: I can afford this brand and the glamorous lifestyle associated with it.

Like any trend, the importance of logos changes throughout the fashion cycle. I recall a particularly lean financial year in grad school when logos were *it*. Forced to choose between food and logos, I Carrie Bradshaw–ed it and chose to go hungry. At the end of the year I had so many plaids, symbols, and letters in my wardrobe that I actually had difficulty dressing. If I stared at myself long enough in the mirrored elevator on my way to class, I could see dolphins swimming or fields of flowers in the patterns. I think I was cured of the logo obsession when I realized that cows have brands on their backsides too.

The logo obsession has become one of the most prevalent fashion errors of our time. The desire to emulate reality television stars, celebrities, and socialites begins with the wardrobe, specifically the logo-laden items. Although this desire seems externally based, the message you wear tells everyone who sees you so much more than that you like Goyard.

Is the Real You Masked by Logos and Labels? A Checklist

- ❏ Do you only buy designer?
- ❏ Do most of your clothes have a logo or a visible label?
- ❏ Do you find it difficult to make outfits because of the logos?
- ❏ Would you buy the items in your closet if they did not have a designer label?
- ❏ Do you enjoy letting people know that you have designer clothes?
- ❏ Do you feel that the logo makes you appear successful?
- ❏ Would you buy a fake designer item just for the visible brand name or design?
- ❏ Do you scour websites and vintage stores for logo-laden items?
- ❏ Do you buy clothes that don't work with your shape or lifestyle just because they're designer?
- ❏ Do you feel insecure when you are not wearing a logo?
- ❏ Do you feel inferior when someone has a "better" or more expensive designer item than you do?
- ❏ When you see someone with this item, do you wish to discard or upgrade your item?

- ☐ Do you believe that a designer label must mean a better-quality garment?
- ☐ Do you like a designer for his or her work or for the mystique associated with the designer's line?
- ☐ Do you spend more than you can afford to have logo items?
- ☐ Do you rent or borrow logo items just so that people will think you can afford them?
- ☐ Have your friends or family suggested that you change your style choices?
- ☐ Do you wish you relied less on logo-laden items?
- ☐ Have you tried to change but been unsuccessful?

If you answered yes to most of these questions, you may have a case of *logo-mania*. This chapter will teach you how to identify your internal reasons for pursuing all things designer, how to find alternatives to logo items, and how to craft your true identity and matching wardrobe without the assistance of a designer's name.

Case Study: How Mary Became Her Own Best Brand

As soon as Mary walked into my office, I knew what her problem was. Wearing clothes that totally ignored practicality and function, she had been blinded by double C's, LV's, and DG's.

"I have all these designer clothes, but I feel that my style is very stale," she said. "It just doesn't have that kick to it. I want to add some spice to my wardrobe, or at least use the pieces I have in a different way."

This woman sitting on the couch across from me was wearing red-soled Louboutin shoes, a black-and-turquoise-beaded Tory Burch logo tunic, and Chanel-emblazoned black leggings, all underneath a beautiful black shearling coat with a fur collar. She was anything but stale—she looked like she was ready to go to a high-end happy hour, not an appointment for styling assistance.

"So, Mary, does this represent your general day-to-day look?"

"Yeah, I usually go for designer looks with some kind of sparkle. I think it's important to dress your best no matter the occasion . . . so here I am."

Mary was kind enough to bring much of her wardrobe to me. After unloading a ton of clothes from her car, we examined her wardrobe piece by piece.

"The first thing I notice, Mary, is the sheer volume of clothes that you have, primarily designer. When did this start?"

Mary's love for high-end clothing, she explained, was cultivated at a very young age in the recesses of her mother's designer closet. Days with her mother were spent feeling the cashmere, silks, and furs hanging from the racks of clothing in her mother's wardrobe. Mary remembered putting her little feet into the hundreds of shoes, in every color, style, fabric, and skin, that lined the floor of the closet. Her most cherished childhood memories were of dressing up and visiting her mother at the upscale clothing store where she worked. Mary can still recall the sound of her mother's heels clacking against the Pergo wood floor of the store.

"So it all started with your mother. She sounds like a spectacular role model for fashion," I said. "When did you begin collecting?"

"I think it started as soon as I had the money to buy it. While in college, I carried on my mother's legacy and began working at a designer retail store. I saw some pretty incredible clothing with even more incredible price tags, but somehow that didn't deter me."

Mary helped impeccably dressed women casually spend thousands of dollars on a pair of pants or a sweater. Soon Mary herself began purchasing the expensive merchandise.

"I really didn't have any business buying these clothes, but looking the part was an important part of the job. I couldn't help these
wealthy women without looking as if I belonged in the same circles
that they came from. I began to slowly acquire the wealthy woman's
wardrobe, but I was far from wealthy."

After seeing enough logos to blind me, we turned to the second
wardrobe mistake, logo-mania. "Mary, I notice not only that you love
designer clothes, but that you love the clothes that explicitly bear
their name. What's going on here?"

Mary was noticeably embarrassed by this question. "Well, it all goes
back to the lack of money thing. Why would I spend an arm and a leg
on something and not want the label on it? I wanted people to know."

As we sifted through the layers and layers of clothes, I struggled
with the strong belief that these pieces should have been featured in
a fashion installment in a museum, not in Mary's closet. "You came
to me because you felt your wardrobe was stale and you had trouble
putting an outfit together. Let's try to make a couple," I suggested.

Mary pulled out some of her favorite pieces and attempted to assemble an ensemble. Ironically, the logos made it nearly impossible
to do so.

"You realize what the problem is, don't you?" Mary shook her
head. "It's tough to make an outfit with all of these patterns. Your logos are working against you."

We needed to find one piece that didn't include a brand-specific
pattern, letter, symbol, or label. A wardrobe requires some blank canvas pieces, and Mary's had none.

Treatment

"Mary," I asked, "if you had all the money in the world, what would
you buy? Would you buy these logo items?"

"Well, if I had all the money in the world, I wouldn't need logos."

"So why do you need them now?"

"Well," she said, and paused. "It makes me feel like I am some-body. I want to look like I am successful. I know how people are treated when they don't look right. My mother told me all about *that.*"

I asked Mary to elaborate. She described what her mother learned from working in retail: "If you want to be someone, you need to dress the part. Whoever said respect is earned was a liar; you just need to dress like you're rich. Why should anyone be treated like anything when they dress like nothing? They don't deserve it."

There was a grain of truth to Mary's words. The outside *does* reflect the inside, but your dressing choices should not alter your value as a human being. In other words, if you aren't wearing expensive clothing, that doesn't mean you don't have worth. Somehow Mary never learned this lesson. She didn't wear logos and designer duds because she liked the designers or liked the pieces. She wore these items to make others value her and ultimately find value within her that she did not believe she inherently deserved.

What Mary didn't tell me at the beginning of our meeting was that through her efforts to look like she had money, she was running out of it. In session it came out that, as she lost more money, her taste for high-end clothing—specifically logo-laden clothing—increased. If she was going to max out her credit cards, forgo buying necessities, and work extra hours to afford expensive items, Mary wanted people to know how much it cost her. Logos are the equivalent of price tags left on clothing. Mary also discovered that her logos compensated for her disappointment in herself, the result of measuring her success by her salary.

I diagnosed Mary with a classic *identity crisis*—using someone else's name to prove her worth. Mary needed to learn who she was by setting and attaining goals, examining her values and beliefs, finding her hidden talents, and understanding her family history, not by wearing certain labels. She also needed to learn what it was like to be judged on her clothes alone.

Stripped

I sent Mary to the mall without her security blanket, the logos to announce her worth. When she headed out stripped of these items, she was not happy. The terrycloth tracksuit and beat-up sneakers she wore to the gym were sure to get her ignored by salespeople . . . and that was the point.

Mary spent the day wandering around high-end stores with a totally low-end look. Just as I had suspected would happen, she was often ignored. I kept her there for an hour or two before deciding it was time to give her some relief.

"What was it like to be judged only by what you wear?"

"It was awful. I didn't feel like a person. The whole thing made me furious. What the hell? What makes them so great? A nice piece of jewelry? A stiletto? A cashmere sweater? I don't think so."

"Mary, I think you got the point. No one should judge *you* based on what you are wearing, so why should you judge anyone else that way? And more importantly, why would you judge yourself using such a faulty measure?" Every time Mary bought a logo item to make herself feel like "someone," she was behaving like the very people who ignored her at the mall. I wanted her to learn that her value lay not in her designer clothes but in her internal qualities.

Now we were able to return to her closet and find what was worth keeping and what needed to go. I assured her that she could find many wonderful clothes that had no logos, were not designer, and would not sink her deeper into debt. This was one idea she was willing to buy.

Reidentification: The Make-Under

After a relatively painless purge of her wardrobe to discard outdated, underworn, over-the-top, and hyper-logo clothing, Mary was prepared to fill in the gaps with some classic pieces that would work with the busy pieces she had in her wardrobe. Stylists often freshen up plain wardrobe items with glam pieces. For example, simple jeans pop with a statement belt, and a plain skirt dressed up with a fancy shoe is plain no more. Mary's wardrobe required a *make-under* in order to freshen up the "stale" pieces. She needed blank canvas clothes to serve as a backdrop for her one-of-a-kind designer pieces.

After examining the items she had left after the cleanup, Mary could go into the stores and find multi-function simple pieces to fill in the gaps. Although she automatically was drawn to the expensive items, I also wanted to show Mary that there were plenty of inexpensive stores where quality clothes could easily be found. Mary wasn't quite sold on the idea and resisted any exploration in the lower-end stores, so I made a deal with her. She would find a look in the high-end store, and I would copy it from a low-end store. Perhaps you've seen this very process on the show *The Look for Less*. Mary's choice of wide-leg jeans, a crisp white shirt, and a wedge heel to go with her Chanel pearl and camellia necklace was easily replicated with items from Express, Limited, Forever 21, and Zara. Through this exercise, Mary discovered that she could choose between the high and low ends and that she had the option to mix and match. You *can* look fabulous on a budget.

After buying a few key pieces, Mary was willing to sift through her old wardrobe again to see if she could make room for the new stuff. When she felt satisfied with her closet, we discussed what to do with her old clothes. We had already thrown away the pieces that weren't salvageable, but there was still plenty there that could find a new closet or be a key piece in someone else's designer collection.

Mary had already landed herself in debt to buy the lifestyle she couldn't afford, so giving away pieces was not an option. I introduced Mary to eBay. Since many of her items were considered vintage or limited edition, Mary would probably be able to auction her pieces off for more than she had paid for them. After a short lesson in the joys of online auctions, Mary was ready to sell her items. During this exercise, Mary also realized that if she simply had to have designer items, she could buy used ones for a fraction of the cost.

After a few weeks of trying out her new wardrobe, selling and buying online, and changing her judgments of others and her faulty perceptions of herself, Mary was ready for a Dr. B follow-up.

"I feel free!"

This is such a consistent response from my clients after I clean out their closet. The paradoxes of letting go to gain control, living with less to feel that you have more, and giving in order to receive are all part of the closet-cleaning experience.

"It's not only the closet that makes me feel free, Dr. B. It's getting rid of the self-judgment. I didn't realize how much my self-judgment chipped away at me until I felt the pain of others doing the same thing to me. It was like a constant running commentary."

Through this experience, Mary learned to identify and reduce that critical voice, which she had internalized from her mother. She acknowledged that when she had a bad day, she began to self-judge. When she countered stress with self-care, her self-judgment ebbed.

"Well, we are all a work in progress, Mary, but I am so happy that you have begun the hardest part," I told her.

Soon Mary realized that, of all the names she wore on her body, her own was the most important. She herself, with nothing more than what she came into the world with, was enough. That alone had the highest value.

Your Turn

Return to Your Senses

From the comfort of our family rooms, we watch the famous, fabulous, and foolish wear beautiful designer clothes that we covet. Whether we're looking at the latest reality star or the newest nominee on the red carpet, we catch a bit of reflected glamour even as we sit in front of our TVs in our bathrobes or curled up in our beds. But watching beautiful people wearing beautiful things in such an accessible way plays tricks on the brain. The more we see television and film stars and celebrities, the more we believe that we can have what they have—or at least, that we ourselves should have what they have. Even though our bank accounts and lifestyles don't match the designer outfits, we buy them anyway. The ole *if-she-can-have-it-so-should-I* trick.

After our brain has convinced us that what we see should be ours, it plays another trick. When we begin to make a habit of buying high-end labels and logo-laden clothing, we become inured to insanely high prices; in psychology we would say that our response becomes extinct. This happened with Mary: each time she purchased an item priced well above her means, her response to that stimuli faded a bit, and eventually her response became extinct.

Certain stimuli elicit *naturally occurring responses*. If I make a loud noise (*stimulus*), you experience shock or fear (*response*). If this stimulus is repeated over and over, however, it no longer elicits a response (*habituation*). Here's a perfect example: if you live near a hospital and hear sirens all day and all night, you eventually tune out the sound. Other stimuli do not elicit a natural response and the response is learned, such as stopping at a red light. When a stimulus no longer elicits a *learned response, extinction* has occurred . . . you blaze through the red light. Since price tags in and of themselves should not elicit any response, the responses we do have to them are learned. The higher the amount on the price tag, the more likely it is that we will respond with shock, and then a decrease in purchasing. As we consistently buy higher-priced items, however, our shock decreases and eventually we reach *sticker shock extinction*. Sound familiar?

So how do we trick our brains into returning to reality? Let's start with *if-she-can-have-it-so-should-I*. Why? Why should you have it? Do you really like the item? Do you really need the item? Does it make sense in your wardrobe? If the answer to any of these questions is no, then you shouldn't buy it.

You know before you buy what it feels like when something is not supposed to be in your wardrobe. Your hands become clammy, your heart races, and your forehead glistens with sweat, but you swipe the card, gritting your teeth behind that fake smile. Don't do it!

Then you need to ask yourself another question. Would you want the item if it were not being worn by a person you obsess over, a person you're jealous of, or a person living the life that you want? If the answer is no, then you shouldn't buy it. Buying something you want just because someone else has it will only lead to losing the desire for it.

What should you do if sticker shock extinction has done severe damage to your wallet? There are several ways to return to your senses. First, shop with someone else, someone who will keep prices in perspective for you. When I was working in retail and selling T-shirts for $500 and jeans for $1,000, I somehow lost my ability to keep prices in perspective. Imagine that! Shopping with friends who would pay no more than $20 for a T-shirt or $50 per pair of jeans helped me find a balance between the ridiculous and the sublime. Second, shopping in lower-end stores or stores that offer deep discounts will show you how much you can get for much less with equal quality. Third, examine the *cost* versus the actual *worth* of the item. For example, a manufacturer can make a plain cotton T-shirt very inexpensively; to pay more than \$10 to \$20 for one is just absurd.

Losing the Logos

I'll admit it: I like really nice things, and sometimes these nice things are logo items. I buy items primarily because I love them, and usually the logo is secondary. But every now and then I like an item because of the logo; if another designer had made it, I probably would not buy it. Getting sucked into the logo cult can happen to anyone, including the most fashionable among us. But help is available!

If you have a case of logo-mania, ask yourself some questions. Why do you like the item? Is it the color, the cut, the function, or the pattern? If it carried another logo, or no logo at all, would you buy it? Finally, is the item a quality piece or a crappy piece with a high-end stamp? These questions will help you find out why you're drawn to logo-laden items as you explore reasons to "buy for the logo" versus "buying for the item."

Quick Tips for Letting Go of Labels

When you use a brand to make up for what you think you lack, your logo obsession has deeper roots. I promise you that using brands this way never works. You experience the initial high of your latest acquisition, but then comes the financial low. And unfortunately, your disappointment does not end with your wallet. You're in for an emotional low as well. In our efforts to shore ourselves up internally by building ourselves up externally, we ultimately let ourselves down and disappointment sets in.

Our country's financial crisis was born of our obsession with keeping up with the Joneses. We buy items we cannot afford in order to create a false life for ourselves. Back in the day, if you didn't have the necessary cash, you didn't make the purchase. Now you can buy now and pay later, but often the cost is far greater than just the monetary cost of financial debt.

If, like Mary, you use logos to "fill the void" and look like you have it all, try reexamining who you would be without all the stuff. Focus on increasing your own value without external supplements. You are enough.

Know who you are: We often lose the ability to be objective about ourselves. Imagine that you are an alien descending on Earth (very dramatic, I know). Imagine that this being can see your physical being, your mental being, your emotional being, and your spiritual being. Taking all of these data points into consideration, what would he say about you? How would he describe you? I am not asking for an opinion here, I am asking for facts. What is true about you?

Have you ever been to an event and had someone else's reaction make you feel totally out of place? At the beginning of the evening you felt spectacular, but one sneer or slight snicker made you feel that you had committed a fashion sin. Who hasn't been in that position? One person, looking us up and down, makes us feel smaller for having what we have and dressing in what we wear. If this person is willing to judge others so harshly, though, imagine how often she judges herself. If you know who you are, such a person will not be able to tear you down by simply projecting her insecurity onto you. You will never feel the need to win the affection of such a person if you are content with what you have under your clothes and under your skin.

Anyone caught up in the pursuit of stuff to make them more this or more that has lost a sense of who they are without the trappings of this world. If this has happened to you, it's time to assess yourself without the stuff—without the job, the car, the house—and identify your worth stripped bare. Having nice things is, well, nice. But seeking out nice things to make you better has the opposite effect. If you know who you are, the latest Birkin bag or Gucci dress won't become a measure of your worth. If you know who you are, then you can sit among people clad in designer duds while wearing a Target top, Old Navy shorts, and Walmart shoes and still feel totally comfortable.

Know what you like: In a world where we are bombarded by the opinions of others, it becomes difficult to tease out your own voice. If we are told that the latest creation from Mr. X is the most innovative, fashion-forward, and coveted collection out there, is that indeed true for you? If the bottom of your shoe weren't painted a blood red, would you buy it for $1,200?

All of us have gotten caught up in the "right" brand, the "right" color, the "right" style that will contribute to our image of success and luxury. In addition to putting a hole in our pocket, choices made according to this criterion may lead us to buy things we don't really want.

In the famous tale by Hans Christian Andersen, "The Emperor's New Clothes," the emperor is told by the tailors that his new pieces are invisible to those who are unworthy. Although he is aware that he is naked, the emperor takes part in the tailors' farce. When he reveals his latest "outfit" to his loyal subjects, it is a child who finally points out that the emperor is naked. Only then do the other subjects agree. Are you like the loyal subjects or the child? Do you want to be part of the herd or have an opinion of your own? Do you actually like what you buy, or are you buying it because you think you are supposed to? Know what you like, and you will know what to wear.

What is your story? We spend so much time consumed by our regrets about the past and the stressors of the present that we often give little thought to our hopes for the future. I fully believe that we create our own story. Yes, obstacles are thrown in our way in the form of illness, difficult relationships, financial hardships, and so on, but we ultimately are the captains of our own ship. Where would you like yours to take you?

If you are caught up in the silliness of attaining external objects, like designer clothes, to make you feel like something, try changing your focus. Forget about empty pursuits and turn your energies toward creating a story for yourself. When you do, the wardrobe will follow. If you want to feel good about yourself, having clothing, food, stuff, and companionship is often not enough; setting a clear life goal and trying to attain it is where the self-esteem comes from. You may never achieve your goal, but your experiences along the way—the efforts, the challenges, the reconsiderations, the changes of direction, the growth—are where you find your value, not in the designer section of Saks.

Become: So you know who you are, you know what you like, and you know the life you want . . . then what are you waiting for? Are you looking for support? Well, guess what? Everyone has enough of their own problems—you need to take care of your own. Are you looking for motivation? Good luck with that one, since motivation comes after you have started. Are you looking for more information? Throw away the self-help books and don't wait another day before taking action toward the vision you have for yourself.

Resist the urge to cloud your vision with the external stuff that you believe will bolster your image. It won't: it is an illusion, and it is not a part of you. You are only tricked into believing that these things will make you more fabulous. Buying from a place of insecurity will only make your insecurity worse, and then you will buy even more. Don't get caught in this trap. If you need to "fast" from shopping, do so. If you need to store your logos, put them away for a while. Only when you have a healthy acceptance of who you are can you cover yourself once again with someone else's name.

Rebalancing a Logo-Heavy Wardrobe

1. *Cease and desist:* Dressing can be difficult when your wardrobe is full of logos. Begin by putting yourself on a logo restriction. When you go shopping, feel free to buy as many designer labels as you would like . . . as long as they are not covered with the logo of the brand.

2. *Purge:* This is the painful part. Look through all of the logo items in your closet. Better yet, throw them on your bed so that you can see the full collection. Pretend that each item is from a no-namer or a designer you do not like. Would you keep the item? If the answer is no, sell or purge it!

3. *Rework and restock:* At this point in the process, the only logo items in your closet should be ones that you love. Mixing and matching these items can overwhelm an outfit as well as the wearer. Having multiple logos in one outfit is a no-no. Having multiple items of the same logo in your outfit is also a no-no. Choose one logo item (a

purse, a sweater, a shoe) and mix it with a simple clean piece (a dark jean, a sweater dress, a cocoon top). If you want to take a greater fashion risk, treat the logo as you would any other pattern—such as layering with florals, stripes, or prints of the same or contrasting hue. When in doubt, have a stylish friend or sales professional help you with this technique.

4. *Picture it:* The camera does not lie. Taking a picture of an outfit helps us see what we really look like. With a picture, we can assess the balance of the outfit, the points of focus, the fit, the effectiveness of the color, and so on. Don't look at the picture immediately—wait a week and then look at your outfit. Often getting some distance from the image will increase your objectivity.

Your outfit will always work when it is chosen for the best version of you. Not for the you who feels fat, not for the you who thinks she's old, and not for the you who hopes logos or designer brands will earn her respect. Remember a time when you felt your best and dress that person. And when someone asks you who designed your outfit, you can proudly exclaim, "I did!"

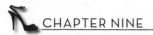

CHAPTER NINE

Getting Back to You

When You Live in Mom Jeans

I know you have seen them. They usually travel in packs. They invade the malls, playing fields, coffeehouses, and schools. From head to toe, the look is unmistakable. Frazzled short hair, cotton turtleneck, pearl earrings, high-waisted or ill-fitting jeans, and dazzling white sneakers. During holidays, they may accessorize with snowball or bunny earrings or a shirt with embroidered images of presents or fireworks. Their affliction is chronic and widespread, usually brought on by bearing children. One day I found myself staring into the eyes of one. The soccer mom.

Jamie came to me exhausted and burned out. As a proud mother of two children, Jamie barely had energy for her full-time job, let alone herself. Like most mothers, Jamie had put her children, husband, and job at the top of her priority list. Sadly, *she* never even made it onto the list. Her wardrobe was a clear indication that Jamie was other-focused.

"Jamie, it sounds like your wardrobe has died and needs to be revived?"

"Oh yeah, it is bad! My husband complains about what I wear all the time. He and my kids say that they are embarrassed by me. I didn't even realize how bad it was until they told me it was."

Jamie's family was more in tune with her wardrobe needs than she was. She continued to tell me that they monitored everything she did. They even told her what her "to-dos" were for the day. I had heard enough and decided to take the plunge into the inner depths of Jamie's incredibly messy closet. What I found wasn't pretty: work sweaters, sweats, T-shirts, elastic, polyester, and washed-out denim.

Jamie went to work wearing the logo of her employer emblazoned on her chest, letting the world know that she supported her company with all of her blood, sweat, and tears. When she wasn't advertising for her employer, Jamie wore sweatshirts, T-shirts, and headbands with the names of her daughters' schools, hobbies, and clubs. Where was Jamie in all of this?

The parts of Jamie that were "employee" and "mother" were reflected in her clothes, but the other parts of her were completely lost. It was time to sit down on the therapist's couch to pull away the layers and find Jamie.

Have You Stopped Dressing for Yourself?
A Checklist

- ☐ Has it been a long time since you purchased something for yourself?
- ☐ Was the item something for your wardrobe?
- ☐ When you go shopping, do you shop for others and not for yourself?
- ☐ When you do shop for yourself, do you feel guilty?
- ☐ Have you given up on looking attractive?

❑ Do you find that you do not have time to dress nicely in
the morning?

❑ Does dressing up take too much energy?

❑ Are you wearing items you once swore you would never wear?

❑ Are your pajamas, lounge, and everyday clothes the same?

❑ Do you choose comfort over style?

❑ Do you dress based on your children's preference?

❑ Do you dress based on your partner's preference?

❑ Do you look at old pictures and miss that woman?

❑ Do you wish you could be her again?

❑ Is it difficult to find "me time"?

❑ When you have it, do you feel guilty?

❑ When you have it, do you think about your family?

❑ Are you unable to sleep because you are thinking about what
you must do for others?

❑ Do you avoid mirrors?

❑ Have you stopped preening activities that you used to engage in,
such as styling your hair or ironing your clothes?

❑ Do you wish that you could dress stylishly?

❑ Are you hesitant to try dressing stylishly because you feel that
you have forgotten how to?

❑ Do you feel out of touch with current fashion trends?

❑ Do you envy women who are able to maintain their style
even with families?

❑ Do you feel that you are long past the point of being stylish?

If you have answered yes to most of these items, you may have
lost yourself to the needs of your family. You cannot give to others
when you don't have anything left for yourself. In this chapter, you
will examine your loss of self, reclaim your identity, and craft a wardrobe to match it.

The Lost Self

Women are raised to nurture. Even if we never become mothers, we tend to be caretakers for friends, families, and significant others. Whether this trait is learned or inherent, we will never really know.

Some women take their caretaker role to the extreme, sacrificing their own needs. The desire to give of one's self completely, I believe, begins with the first dating relationship. Many of us have our first dating experience in adolescence, a time when we are learning not only about our bodies, our minds, and our emotions but about who we are in relation to a partner.

When you were a child, your parents dressed you. As you got older, you learned that you too could make choices about what to wear, but your decision to wear a pink tutu to church was probably overturned. Finally, after many years of fashion dependence, you attained fashion independence. You had the right to make any fashion mistakes you wanted. Then you began dating.

At first you wore what you liked: T-shirts, jeans, and sneakers. Then your new boyfriend began dropping little comments about his appreciation of girls in dresses. When you went out to dinner, you saw him noticing the petite brunette in the corner of the room in the flouncy pink number . . . while you sat across from him in your button-down and khakis. Insecurity set in. Whether real or imagined, you became afraid. How could you hook this guy when your life looked like it was going to be filled with petite brunettes sitting in the corners of your relationship? Something had to change. That something would be you.

That is when the sacrifice of self began. You swore off the comfortable clothes you loved for clothes you *thought* your boyfriend would like. You bought an armload of dresses in every girlie color under the rainbow, you ignored your sore knees and wore the four-inch heels, and you even spackled on some makeup. Would he notice? Would you keep him? And then it happened.

"Wow, you got a new look going on."

Startled, you blink your eyes rapidly. "Sooo, do you like it?"

"Yeah, you look great. It just looks different."

"What do you mean? I thought you would like it. You told me you like dresses, and here I am wearing one. What the heck? What do you want?"

Caught off guard, he collects his thoughts. "You, I want you. Is this you?"

Ah, the irony of it all. You're trying to give your man what you think he wants, but what he really wants, what he was initially attracted to, and what keeps him around, is *you!*

If we are lucky enough to have a positive first experience, the trust and mutual respect in an early relationship allows us to feel free to maintain all that we are, both good and bad. Even with the most wonderful man, however, we may be unable to conquer our desire to please. We like the music he likes, go where he wants to go, clean his apartment for him, or spend time exploring his hobbies. Initially, our man may appreciate our desire to become everything he would like, but eventually the new car smell of the relationship wears off. After the infatuation wears off, we either throw off the mask and show our partner who we really are or sacrifice our own identity to plunge even deeper into his world. Depending on the man, the decision to give up who we are will either scare him off or attract him. Regardless of men's reactions, becoming someone other than ourselves in order to find love happens more often than it should.

Often this process begins very quietly. Losing ourselves in a relationship starts with very small decisions and an eagerness to please, and before we know it, active decisions have become mindless habits. We often only become aware of our loss of self after the relationship breaks apart. The tendency to lose the self doesn't end with our first loves. I have met many wives and mothers who feel that they no longer know who they are other than someone who meets their husband's and children's needs. With the departure of the children for college or the approach of retirement, they finally are faced with the truth that the person they were has been stuffed under the bed with the kiddie toys. So many of the clients I work with need to be reintroduced to themselves.

Coming back to who they are must start with acknowledging that they lost something. Then they must decide who they are now and how they lost themselves in the first place.

One of the first places I look to find the lost self is in the closet. It is here where the forgotten past lies. It is here where the present cannot be escaped. It is here where the future has endless possibilities.

Case Study: The Importance of Dressing for Jamie and Only Jamie

So back to Jamie—who was she? Ever organized, she didn't have anything in her closet from years past that could help me see her style metamorphosis. "What might I have found in your old closet?" I asked.

"Well, I certainly didn't live in jeans, T-shirts, and button-downs, I'll tell you that much," she laughed. "I wore soft fabrics, like silk and chiffon. Totally not mommy appropriate! I loved anything that showed off my legs and arms, which, thank God, still look good. Although I really don't show them off because I want to look like a mom, and I don't think the sexy thing works. Not to mention my kids and hubby would kill me."

We went through the clothes and saved the must-haves, such as the pieces Jamie would need to wear to work. We also kept the clothes she wanted to wear for her children's games and trips to the gym. The rest, such as the embroidered capri pants, stretchy jeans, and printed T-shirts were given to the local thrift store.

"Jamie, is there anything here that speaks to the person you were before the children and husband?"

"No, not really. I guess my date night clothes are the only thing that comes close, that have some femininity. The weird thing is, I almost feel uncomfortable tapping into my feminine side with a husband and children, but what I am wearing right now doesn't work for them either."

"So why has your wardrobe become this?" I said, pointing to the pieces on the floor.

"I feel really weird wearing all these pretty things. When I try to, my husband and children give me *the look*."

"So when you try to return to who you were, there is resistance, but when you try to accommodate your family with your current look they are not satisfied?"

"Yes, I feel that I am letting them down."

"Like you are supposed to be one thing for them, but you are another for yourself."

"Yes, yes. I want to be the mother, the wife, but that look is not the look for Jamie. Rather than upsetting them, I stick to the mother/wife look and forget Jamie."

This is quite common, even among those whose families have brought them in for help. On the one hand, the family knows that you need assistance and they want you to improve. On the other hand, when you are working through a process toward healing, your family is uncomfortable with the change. They resist the change in you because they are resisting the shifts in family dynamics, roles, and interactions and the new expectations and needs. Jamie's family needed some time to accept the changes she was initiating, but with her understanding and assurance, they would do it!

"You don't want to lose yourself," I told her. "There is a way to be both yourself and the mother and wife in your family, if that's what matters to you. Before we even begin to alter your wardrobe, we need to connect who you are now with who you were then. Who are you now?"

"Well, isn't it obvious? I am a devoted wife and mother."

"And who were you in the past?"

"Remembering who I was is much harder."

"Jamie, take out your old albums, yearbooks, and scrapbooks. Show me who you were."

While searching through boxes of old photographs, Jamie was reminded of her life before marriage and children. There was a time when she enjoyed going to the beach and designing interiors, and there was even a time when she would pack her bag at a moment's notice to travel to Paris, Milan, or Argentina and return with boxes of the local fashions. These interests, like the pictures, were buried far away and forgotten.

Could Jamie still be a free spirit with a husband and children? There was one way to find out. I asked, "Jamie, could you tell me who you are now? Tell me what you do. What does your life look like?"

Jamie's best description of her life was found within the pages of her daily planner. Upon examination, I found that most of the time in Jamie's schedule that was not given to work was given to her children. Certainly she didn't have as much free time as she once had, but accommodations could be made to find a suitable balance.

"Okay, let's look at what you've got. I see a lot of time taken for work in the morning, and your afternoon is given to your children's activities. I am seeing some free time in the early evening, and I see that on the weekends, when your children are gone, you do have some free blocks. It's important to schedule time to unwind, nap, and do nothing. I also want to schedule some time twice a week for you to pursue something you love."

I am all for parents spending time with their children and with each other. If you are going to have children, it is your responsibility to raise them. Time spent helping your children with their academics, hobbies, and social interactions is part of your job as a parent. That being said, you cannot be a healthy parent if you have depleted your resources through overscheduling and lack of self-care.

After blocking out chunks of time for Jamie, we were ready to fill in the slots with activities. At first, Jamie was unable to list activities or interests that were not directly linked to her children or husband. It took some thought, but eventually Jamie found time in her day, identified her areas of interest, made a plan to pursue her hobbies, and obtained her family's support in helping her properly use her well-deserved "me time." She purchased interior design books to study, scheduled trips to flea markets and antique shops, and took over the research and planning for family trips to the places she had always enjoyed.

With renewed energy and excitement about her own life, Jamie was finally prepared to tackle the mommy gear in her closet and the resistance from her family.

Reidentification

People are not one-dimensional creatures. Being a wife and a mother is just one component of some women's identity. Unfortunately, many choose to ignore the other aspects of the self, relegating them to dark corners of their person. Those pieces of the self become lost or underdeveloped.

Part of enabling Jamie to see herself from a full 360-degree perspective was reintroducing her to her former activities and passions.

She was more than a wife and mother—she was also a sister, daughter, friend, flirt, beachcomber, traveler, stargazer, and dreamer. Over the years, as she had lost those pieces of herself, her wardrobe had followed. A wardrobe that had once been soft and feminine turned into an asexual mommy wardrobe.

As Jamie slowly uncovered the person she thought she had lost, she became tired of eyelet, crazy quilt–inspired patterns, and buttons in the shape of fruits and flowers. These items no longer made sense for her. As though she were wearing the costume of another character, Jamie was not the person her clothes told her she should be. After an internal remake, Jamie could find the clothes that spoke to the "new" Jamie—the new Jamie being a seamless combination of the old Jamie in a new set of circumstances.

The old Jamie wanted sexy and feminine clothes, but her new set of circumstances required that her clothes be appropriate for PTA meetings and soccer games. The old Jamie wanted to wear silky fabrics, but the new Jamie needed low-maintenance clothing. The old Jamie was bony with a flat stomach, but the new Jamie was much more muscular with a slight baby pooch. As we shopped together, we worked toward a compromise between the two Jamies.

We looked for clothing with clean and structured lines for her figure, offset by soft colors to increase femininity. And we made a deal: the logo sweatshirts and university tees were for game days only. These were traded in for boatneck tops and washable silk blouses. Her colored corduroy pants with embroidered critters and her clogs were exchanged for forgiving palazzo pants and chunky woven wedges. After her life-changing style transformation, Jamie became not just any mother but one hot mama!

The final step in her reidentification was to introduce Jamie's new and improved look to her family. For her, this was the most critical part of the makeover. I believed that if her family did not accept

Jamie's new look, she would go back to her old wardrobe. Families, especially children, may have difficulty when the mother is physically changed. The younger the child, the more likely he or she is to believe that a new haircut or clothing style means an internal change in Mommy. (One of my earliest memories of my brother is of his reaction to my mother cutting her long hair into a chin-length bob. He had difficulty making sense of the "new mommy" and believed that the changes in her went beyond the hairstyle.)

Fear of change is a factor in our understanding of *constancy* in cognitive development. If I remove an object from the sight of a young child, he believes that the object no longer exists; as he gets older, he learns that the object may still exist even if he can't see it. Applying this theory closer to home, when a mother leaves for work, her child may initially cry because he believes that she is never coming back. Eventually, as the mother returns each time, he learns that she is always coming back.

Jamie's husband and children were struggling with constancy! In the past when Jamie attempted to change her look, they believed that the mother and wife they loved was also gone, even though she remained. As part of her makeover process, Jamie needed to be prepared for initial rejection of her new look by her husband and children— even though they were the ones who requested it!—but with time they would realize that Jamie the mother and wife they knew and loved was still there, just wrapped in a different package. They would also realize that as she took time for personal development and self-discovery, the fundamentals of her person would remain available to them. Only time would tell whether Jamie's family would feel comfortable with the changes she was making.

A month after Jamie's makeover, I decided to check in to find out how Jamie and her family were handling the transition.

"Well, Dr. B, the first two weeks were pretty rough. My family loved the way I looked, but they still said they missed the 'old me.'

Per your suggestion, I consistently reassured them that I was still the same person, just looking better."

"And the internal changes?"

"Interestingly enough, they were able to handle really well the time I found for myself, the hobbies I pursued, and the improvements in my mood and ability to relax. They actually encouraged me to do the things I love because they see a happier mommy and wife. The hardest part was the external piece."

"That makes sense, since the external piece is the most concrete, obvious, and measurable," I noted. "They also may not see how they benefit from it. The internal changes are more difficult to tally, but they directly benefit the quality of the relationship they have with you. Now, how are you feeling?"

"I really thought I would feel like a new person. I actually don't. I feel like the best version of the old me. And as you said, I feel like 'the old me in a new situation.' I felt that I had kept that part of me secret for so long, and it felt so relieving to reveal it."

Your Turn

The most common complaint I hear from mothers and wives is, "I have lost myself," to which I say, "Then go find yourself!" It is your primary parental obligation. If you are a mother or wife, making time for yourself may seem to be impossible, but it is essential that you do it. It will make you a better version of you. I always use the oxygen mask on the airplane analogy. Before helping another person with their oxygen mask, *you* must put on your own mask first.

Taking time for yourself does not mean abandoning your responsibilities. Taking time for yourself means using ten minutes of free time to look through your favorite magazine, have a cup of coffee, meditate, stretch, go outside, paint your nails, or even pick out an attractive outfit for the day. Take full advantage of your free time to use it for your-self. As your children get older and require less of you, require more of your own attention. Ultimately, if you lose yourself in motherhood or marriage, you are lost to your family as well.

One of the easiest forms of self-care is dressing well. Even if your schedule is overwhelming, looking good should take only five minutes if you have a well-constructed wardrobe. And the time you invest in put-ting on an attractive outfit multiplies a hundred-fold in the reward. The effect of wearing a nice cotton dress with chic sandals, which take less time to put on than sweats and sneakers, lasts throughout the day. In the morning, use the five minutes when you dress to find quiet and relax-ation. Then, as the day progresses, you will feel pretty as you catch your-self in the mirror, the confidence you exude will be palpable, others will be more likely to treat you with the same care you have given yourself, and your children and husband may even notice that you look fantastic. As your confidence strengthens, you are more likely to continue dressing well. This cycle between you, your actions, and the environment can be best described using psychologist Albert Bandura's *reciprocal determin-ism.** He proposed that the interplay between you, your behaviors, and the environment are multidirectional, equally impacting each other.

Becoming a Role Model Beyond the Closet

Initially, discovering who you are is critical to your development. Knowing your boundaries, beliefs, likes, and dislikes as they surface in your relationships with others is the second component of self-discovery. The final step in self-discovery is having someone look to you to discover who they are. This is quite a heavy responsibility, and

---

* A. Bandura, *Social Foundations of Thought and Action: A Social Cognitive Theory* (Englewood Cliffs, NJ: Prentice-Hall, 1986).

one that parents especially must take seriously. Your children are watching you to understand themselves.

Parents want their children to feel good about themselves, to take care of themselves, and to develop high self-esteem. The parents who come to me for advice on how to help their children achieve these things are the same parents who ask why their offspring, in spite of parental love and support, feel so bad about themselves. The answer may lie with how the parents value themselves. A mother who constantly makes comments about her "big ole pooch" or her "bubble butt" wonders why her nine-year-old daughter hates her body and wants to lose weight. A workaholic father wonders why his child takes hours to get her homework done because she can "never get it quite right." Sound familiar?

You can talk all you want about the importance of your children acknowledging and loving who they are, but if *you* are not living this message, your children will not buy it. Children are intelligent and sophisticated creatures who learn through imitation and modeling. They will always copy your behaviors before listening to what you say.

When it comes to identity formation, a daughter watching you sacrifice who you are to please another is learning that wonderful skill from you! To teach her to respect her own boundaries, beliefs, values, and even her preference for five-inch platform heels, you must be prepared to protect your own boundaries, beliefs, values, and preferences.

She will notice when you take time for yourself, especially when it comes to dressing. Your daughter will model her behavior from your behavior and pay attention to your efforts, not empty words, to improve your appearance. Mothers, attend to the messages you are sending your girls. Your actions will become hers when she is a mother. She needs to see that her mother cares about herself and her appearance.

A ROLE MODEL ON AND OFF THE RUNWAY

My mother has done it all and looked great doing it. This is a woman who painted our entire basement while wearing a silk suit. Like her mother, my mother has always worn heels, chic ensembles, jewelry, and full makeup. Jeans, flats, and sneakers have never entered my mother's closet. Although last year she finally bought a pair of jeans . . . with *beading!*

In one of my earliest memories, I was sitting under my mother's dressing table in our first house. Shielded from the bright vanity lights, I watched her brush green shadow around her striking dark eyes, fasten on her colorful lizard-skin heels, and place tortoiseshell combs in her black hair. Until this point, I had only thought of her as the one who fed me, changed my diaper, danced with me, and rocked me to sleep. But through those small, seemingly insignificant preening actions, I realized that if she had other components to her being I must have them too, and that these aspects of self also needed care. This was a lesson that all the talking in the world would never have conveyed. In the warm glow of the mirror, my mother peeked under her table, spotted me, and swept me up into her arms. Even though I was very young, I remember being thankful that I could share this surreal moment with the beautiful woman who chose to be my mother.

Quick Tips for Owning Your Identity

Know Your History

Inside: You are part of something greater than yourself; the line of your existence does not begin and end with you. You are a chapter of a larger story, beginnings and endings being merely temporal constructs.

You are the physical expression of a DNA recipe that long preceded you, that was millennia in the making. Your internal experience, including your soothing methods, interpersonal interactions, and emotional reactions, is not just born from you. It is created from your environment, particularly from the impact of your caretakers and your peer interactions. Really knowing who you are does not begin with yourself. You must dig a little deeper through the layers to find out the history of your being.

Find your history by speaking with family members and friends. Examine the old photos, letters, and journals. If your past was a difficult one, work with a professional who can help you process it and find closure. If you have no history of your past owing to adoption, displacement, or another trauma, see what you can find out through investigation. If this is too painful, work with a professional to find closure in your past.

Outside: Just as you can learn so much by examining what you choose to wear each day, you can also learn a great deal from examining the attire of those around you. Dig into the old family photos and analyze what you see. I have little memory of my grandfather, but I learned about him by looking at his pictures. He was always in either a suit or outdoor attire—an executive and a sporting man. I learned that he enjoyed a challenge, thrived on competition, and loved interacting with people. My mother's desire to be with people and excel at challenges made more sense. My own desire to seek out challenges became clearer. All it took was seeing a few pictures of my grandfather in an album.

You can do even better than pictures. My love for the psychology of dress grew from my first experience in my grandmother's closet. It was there that I learned the most about her, which led to discoveries about my mother, which illuminated my own self-knowledge. Use external pieces from important people in your life, such as clothing, jewelry, and shoes, to learn more about them—and ultimately discover yourself!

Know Who You Are

Inside: I work with many adolescent females, who are my favorite patient population. One of my favorite activities I use with them is what I call the *identity box:* I write personal questions for a teenage patient on slips of paper, fold them, put them in the box, and then ask her to pull the questions out of the box one by one and answer them. Through this activity, she teaches me who she is and learns about herself, but more importantly, she learns how little self-knowledge she actually has. She is forced to search for her identity when the identity box questions are unanswerable.

You don't have to be a teenager to do something similar. One of my many harebrained ideas was to compete for an opportunity to have a talk show on the OWN network. Although my schedule did not allow me to even consider actually applying for the show, I still took the time to answer the questions on the application. One of the application requirements was to fill out a thick packet of questions about my dreams, accomplishments, weaknesses, talents, and so on. I thought I was pretty knowledgeable about myself—I was a shrink, for God's sake—but as I struggled for answers I realized that I wasn't.

There are many opportunities out there to find similar activities. If you have ever filled out an online dating profile, such as Match or eHarmony, you know that they require self-exploration. You can also try the book *The Hard Questions: 100 Essential Questions to Ask Before You Say "I Do"* by Susan Piver.* Although meant for couples, it

---

* S. Piver, *The Hard Questions: 100 Essential Questions to Ask Before You Say "I Do"* (New York: Tarcher/Putnam, 2000).

can be great for just you. Another option is to write your obituary, as though who you hope to be someday is telling you who you are now.

Outside: The internal work is only part of the self-discovery process. What you present to yourself and the world can also teach you about who you are. Nothing is better than looking through old pictures and seeing what you looked like in an earlier era. Many of us cringe when we see our '80s moment, complete with leggings, scrunchie, tight rolled jeans, and teased perm. Some of us had the grunge '90s moment, the '70s disco moment, the emo moment of the 2000s, and so on. We can learn through our attire who we were and how we have come to our present life just by looking at what we wore.

Your style speaks so much to your internal state and resultant lifestyle. If you felt like crap about your body, you probably covered it up. If you felt like your life was free and full of adventure, your clothes spoke to this internal confidence. If you were struggling financially, you wore vintage. When you got your first job, you rocked the suit.

Even examining your style transitions can show you the larger developmental changes you made. At the time in my life when I found internal confidence, my look found variation. In pictures I see images of white button-downs, jeans, and cable knit crewnecks changing into fashion-forward dresses and high-fashion shoes. When I met the love of my life, my wardrobe found color and figure-flattering shapes. My shoes grew a few inches with each date. Look at your style evolution to find important biographical landmarks. Trust me—they are there.

Take a Risk

Inside: It has been said that we never really know who we are until we have been faced with a challenge. When we ask, "What would I do if? . . ." we never really know if our hypothetical response would match our actual response. I would never harm someone, but if someone hurt a loved one of mine, I might not be able to resist retribution.

No one wants to be put in a difficult situation, such as losing a loved one, filing for bankruptcy, getting divorced, or losing a job. But it's these very situations that teach us the most about who we are. We learn about our limitations, our strengths and weaknesses, and how resourceful and self-reliant we are; we also learn the true depth of our friendships.

I know that life is stressful enough without the additional stressors that come with discovering self-identify, but self-created risks do offer smaller-scale opportunities to stretch, grow, and learn who we really are. It is through running a marathon, taking on a public speaking gig, deciding to take a new class, or dumping a loser that we discover what we are made of.

Outside: When we are repeatedly faced with a novel stimulus, we become habituated to its effects. We no longer attend to something that would once have annoyed us, such as the sound of construction outside our window every day all day. Now it's time to apply this idea to your look. One of the easiest ways to explore your identity is to change your look. What you wear can shift your perception of yourself and others' perceptions of you in a positive or negative way.

Although who you are and the demands of your life will determine how often you can change your look, I would suggest that you aim to do it at least once a year. Like a birthday or anniversary, a new look can become part of your "new year/new you" routine. Even if you don't want to make a yearly commitment to change your look, you can still take an internal inventory each year. Do you find that you look the same in pictures from year to the next? Are you finding that getting ready in the morning has become rote? Do you avoid mirrors? Then it's time for a change.

You know what happens when you take a risk. Your heart races, your palms sweat, and you grit your teeth . . . but you're smiling! Taking a risk, even if it is just with your look, can take you out of a rut. Wear a bright color, throw out the girdle, or show a little leg. Do something that makes you scared and excited! Your mirror will thank you.

Mommy Wardrobe Quick Tips

If you are short on time and heavy on tasks, follow these tips to make your life as easy as possible.

- Stain-resistant is a must. If you have young children, don't buy anything for yourself that you can't wash. If you must wear high-maintenance pieces, save time by using a home delivery dry cleaner. Carry a stain removal pen and wet naps in your purse or glove compartment so that you are always prepared for life's many messes. Patterned fabrics are wonderful at camouflaging stains!
- Many designers offer machine-washable items. Do your research—check online and in the store for wash-and-go items. Find a knowledgeable salesperson in a major department store to help you identify brands that specialize in washable styles.
- Don't waste time with wrinkles. Find items that are wrinkle-resistant. Many fabrics, even those that require ironing, can stay wrinkle-free if you hang them immediately after the dryer cycle ends.
- Think stretchy. You don't want to be constricted when you are running here and there, picking up and putting down children. If you are uncomfortable with your weight or have problem areas, stretchy fabrics can conceal, especially when gathered.

- Forget the fuss. Keep it simple when you dress. Forget the five-inch stilettos, forgo the layers of bangles, and give up the ties and clasps. Find items that slip on and off with ease, don't interfere with your activities, and keep you comfortable.

- Don't forget the sexy. You are still a woman! Wear something that makes you feel beautiful—maybe a bright color, a spectacular earring, a metallic knit, a patterned stocking, or a fitted-and-flared day dress. Play up your legs, show off your arms, rock that bum, or flash a little cleavage.

- Take a risk. I have suggested that you play it safe most of the time for ease, but sometimes you need to step out on the fashion ledge. Look through fashion magazines and online style blogs for inspiration. Pick out two to three looks and try them out on date night or a day out with the girls.

Throughout our lives we wear many hats. Student, daughter, employee, boss, athlete, artist, wife, and mother. The common thread running through all of these roles is you. Regardless of your situation, do not lose yourself in your busy life—or in your closet!

Now What?

Here we are at the end of the journey. If you have taken anything from this book, I hope it is that your closet contains so much more than your clothes. It holds your story. In this small unassuming space, you can find where you have been, where you are, and where you need to go.

Through this analysis, discover the changes you need to make to create a better life. When you take the time and make the effort to alter one area of your life, such as the contents of your closet, improvement in other areas soon follows. You are worth taking care of, whether in mind, body, or wardrobe.

One of my favorite quotes is from Auntie Mame. A woman who had a full life and a wardrobe to match, she exclaimed: "Life is a banquet, and most poor sons of bitches are starving to death. Live!" Don't be the person who walks around starving—be the person who hungers for life and swallows it whole . . . but be sure to dress well for the meal!

Appendix:
Do-It-Yourself Wardrobe Analysis

By now you have read this book and examined the case studies, both of which I hope gave you some helpful information, motivation, and inspiration to make wonderful changes in your wardrobe and life. Although the methods I use do require real psychological training, you can use my steps to try making this transformation for yourself. You might even team up with a friend or support group to see where this InsideOut transformation leads.

Here are the five steps of a wardrobe analysis that will lead to your very own InsideOut makeover.

Wardrobe Analysis:
1. Examination
2. Formulation
3. Change
4. Exploration
5. Future

Examining what you have and why you have it: Begin by blowing the top off your wardrobe and dig in. Look first for fashion patterns. Do your clothes tend not to fit properly? Are they age-inappropriate? Do you never wear them, or are they out of date?

The second part of this step is to make the connection between your clothing patterns and psychological reasons for them. The reasons for these patterns may include being stuck in a life rut, having body image issues, feeling aging fears, experiencing arrested development, falling into regression, and living an unfulfilled life. Also examine the emotions each piece of your wardrobe draws from you.

Formulating the wardrobe and the life that you want: This step has two parts. The first is to think about your life goals. Who do you want to be? Where do you want to go? What do you want to accomplish? What do you want to change? And here's my absolute favorite question: how will you know you are living a fulfilling life?

The second part is to formulate the wardrobe you would like to have. Examine if your wardrobe matches the life and style that you desire. This is the part of the process where you can examine a style file for inspiration. You can also decide which of your wardrobe pieces are keepers and what items your wardrobe needs, based on your body type, color palette, lifestyle, and budget

What will you purge? What will you keep? What will you buy? Making actual changes, not surprisingly, is often the most difficult and exciting step. Change is hard to discuss and plan for, but implementing it doesn't need to become an impossible task. It is during this step that you fill in the gaps between where you are and where you want to go, in terms of both your life goals and your wardrobe goals. As you've learned in this book, the two kinds of goals are strongly connected and mutually reinforcing. If you cannot buy into the need to make and carry out a plan, it simply will not happen. So as you plan the steps of the changes you're going to make, you must carefully examine your reasoning behind each change.

After you make a life and wardrobe plan, it's time to purge, shop, and fill your planner with your psychological "homework!"

Exploring what just happened: The initial changes—purging your closet, making a plan, shopping, starting new activities—can feel wonderful at first. The next day or week might be a different story. Shifts in your dress and your life can become overwhelming, scary, and tiring. A check-in and a debriefing are always critical in any makeover.

Ask yourself some of the questions I pose to my clients right after our sessions. What were you feeling before, during, and after the makeover? Which parts feel easy and which parts do you find yourself resisting? How do you feel in your new clothes? How are others responding to you? How are you handling those responses? How are you responding to yourself?

Check in with yourself a second time after a week or two. You're likely to discover that your responses to these questions have changed. In fact, as happens with most of my clients, you may be feeling more comfortable by then and maybe even feeling "lighter."

What's next? In the final step, determine what items you still need in your closet to match your lifestyle. This is also the time for you to generate a future life plan, spelling out your short-term and long-term goals and generating clear steps to accomplish each one. I also strongly suggest that you craft an emergency plan for handling any problems you can foresee in the future.

Wardrobe Analysis

The Examination:
What do you have and why do you have it?

External
- Examine the contents of your wardrobe
- Examine the patterns of your dress behavior

Internal
- Examine the underlying reasons for your wardrobe choices
- Assess the emotional response your wardrobe elicits

The Formulation:
What wardrobe and what life do you want?

External
- Identify your ideal look to match your newly formulated life

- Assess your body type
- Assess your color palette
- Assess your lifestyle
- Assess your budget

Internal
- Where are you in your life?
- Where do you want to go?

Making Changes:
What items will you purge, buy, or keep? Why?

External
- Clean out your closet
- Identify your wardrobe needs
- Acquire the clothing and accessory items you need to fill the gaps

Internal
- Determine what will facilitate your style transition
- Implement your action plan to achieve your goals

The Exploration: What just happened?

External
- Assess your wardrobe change
- Examine your external identity shift

Internal
- Examine your emotional experience of your external changes
- Process your internal changes

The Future: What's next?

External
- What items do you need to buy now?
- What items do you need to buy in the future?

Internal
- What are your goals for the future?
- What internal obstacles to achieving these goals do you foresee?
- What are some strategies to remove those obstacles?

Sample Wardrobe Analysis

Mrs. X is a thirty-something who has returned to school. Since she was last in school, she has experienced serious medical problems, suffered financial difficulties, and gained weight.

The Examination: What do you have and why do you have it?

Mrs. X has oversized items in her closet that she uses to hide her body and the weight she has gained from medication; more specifically, she is self-conscious about her large chest.

Her closet also includes inexpensive, lower-quality items she has bought because paying medical bills—and now school tuition—has left her financially strapped.

Self-conscious because of how her medical problems, she believes, make her stand out, she wears the worn-out and stained pieces in her closet because she doesn't want to draw further attention to herself.

Her clothing pieces are not interchangeable because she has difficulty mixing and matching, doesn't know how to put together outfits, and is insecure about "making a mistake" and "standing out because of it."

Her wardrobe consists of casual pieces only, such as sweats and T-shirts, and her work uniform.

Mrs. X is stuck in a rut and uncomfortable with transitioning.

The Formulation:
What wardrobe and what life do you want?

Mrs. X wants to enjoy activities with her friends before starting school.

She wants to strengthen her social skills, especially with an eye toward meeting new friends in school.

She wants to be less anxious about standing out because of her
medical condition.

She wants to find "grown-up clothes" and classic items "with a twist."

She wants to wear casual items that are comfortable and soft but
not sloppy.

She needs items that will provide coverage for her chest but will still
be attractive.

Making Changes: What will you purge?
What will you keep? What will you buy?

Mrs. X decided to examine her social difficulties by practicing and
implementing new skills, such as reading nonverbal cues,
identifying her own nonverbal signals, posturing, eye contact,
walk, introduction skills, open-ended questions, continuing
conversations, and ending conversations.

She created a social to-do list, including plans to host a party with
friends before the start of school and then gatherings on weekends
and during school breaks.

She created a social networking presence online to increase her contact
with her friends.

Through role-play, she learned how to explain her medical condition to
strangers when they stared or asked questions.

To save herself money in the long run, she began to buy higher-priced
items of better quality.

To help her be less self-conscious about her weight gain, she found
clothing that fit at the narrowest part of her body and floated away
at the wider part (the baby-doll silhouette).

She learned to choose soft and comfortable fabrics (cotton jersey) that
would make her feel comfortable but not sloppy.

She bought jewel-tone colors that would help her stand out in a crowd
without being too loud.

She bought appropriate foundation garments for her chest, and for
better coverage she switched to wearing deep-V tops with pretty
camis underneath.

She learned to create outfits without making "mistakes" by choosing clothing with a theme—jewel tone colors, a fit and flowy silhouette, or classic shapes with a point of interest such as gathers, pleats, or weave.

She learned to identify classic pieces and to accessorize with trendier pieces to feel more adult.

The Exploration: What just happened?

Overexposure

Mrs. X learned that if you're uncomfortable with certain areas of your body, such as your lower body (this is true for most women), then maximize the parts you love, such as your waist or arms.

She learned how to balance her silhouette. Since her upper body was larger than her lower body, she anchored her body with a chunky heel or boot. By the same principle, someone with narrow shoulders and wider hips could wear a cap-sleeve shirt, a top gathered at the shoulder, or a well-structured blazer.

She identified the origin of her body concerns and sorted out the real ones from those based on misperception.

Concerns About Cost

Mrs. X downgraded the items in her closet so that she was still wearing them, but for more casual occasions.

She began using multifunctional clothing, such as tops that could go from a day at the park to an evening at the movies.

She bought accessories to dress up or dress down her multifunction clothing, such as fun and colorful plastic bangles for the day and gold or silver bangles for the evening.

She bought high-quality classic clothing that she could wear for years and learned to measure the true cost of an item with this formula: total cost equals the price divided by the number of uses.

Getting a Fresh Start Going Back to School

When Mrs. X's social interactions improved, she got involved in more activities and her general mood improved as well. Her clothing reflected and reinforced this internal experience.

She was dressing in a way that made that all-important good first impression by showing others that she valued herself.

She became more comfortable with drawing attention to herself, and when she was not, at least she was less likely to try to fade into the background.

As someone struggling with medical concerns, she especially deserved the chance to dress well in order to pamper herself and to enjoy the "treat" of wearing clothes from a wonderful and rewarding wardrobe.

The Future: What's next?

Mrs. X will take a class to improve her public speaking skills.

She will join clubs she's interested in at school to meet new people in a safe environment.

In addition to pursuing her hobbies and interests, she will invite others to join her.

She will dress trendy but still classic by buying skinny jeans to tuck into her boots and to wear with flats.

She will help herself feel "more adult" by buying a black skirt to wear with all of her tops and her boots, flats, or heels on dressier occasions.

For maximum coverage and support, she will wear a nude-colored, lightly padded bra.

She will buy accessories as needed, including hats, gloves, tights, leggings, bangles, earrings, and clutches.

Index